In 1924, Michael J. Scott, M.D., announced in a Montana newspaper that he had a new, effective cure for cancer based on an antiserum against certain bacteria associated with cancer—and he proved it!

Using the same approach, other doctors in the East cured hundreds of men, women, and children in the next twenty years.

In the meantime, a number of qualified scientists in Europe and the United States have added evidence upon evidence of the role of bacteria in cancer. This is not to be confused with the propaganda about viruses and cancer we have heard so much about.

As a result of their bacterial work, we now have a scientifically sound basis for new therapies, new diagnostic tools, and, above all, a preventive vaccine against all cancer!

But you have not heard anything about this major breakthrough in newspapers, magazines, books, or TV news with the exception of a national TV presentation by NBC Nightly TV News in 1977.

Why?

Because the medical-industrial complex has erected an iron curtain of dogma around cancer research.

Because, in effect, there is a conspiracy of silence and repression in the world of medical research.

And this book dares to challenge that conspiracy!

When you read it, you will want to do something about it!

THE CANCER CONSPIRACY

ROBERT E. NETTERBERG
and
ROBERT T. TAYLOR

PINNACLE BOOKS NEW YORK

THE CANCER CONSPIRACY

An original Pinnacle Books edition, published for the first time anywhere.

First printing, September 1981

ISBN: 0-523-41466-8

Printed in the United States of America

PINNACLE BOOKS, INC.
1430 Broadway
New York, New York 10018

Truth never comes into the world but like a bastard, to the ignominy of him that brought her forth.

—John Milton, *Areopagitica*

E pur si muove—But it does move!

—Attributed to Galileo after recanting his assertion that the earth moves around the sun.

Two roads diverged in a wood, and I—
I took the one less traveled by
And that has made all the difference.

—Robert Frost, "The Road Not Taken"

To all scientists who are devoting their lives to the conquest of cancer.

Acknowledgments

We wish to thank the following for their efforts to bring this material to public notice:

Roy Neal
NBC News
Los Angeles, California

Bill Wheatley
Senior Producer, NBC News
New York, New York

Paul Harvey, Chicago, Illinois

Rick Foote
Staff Writer
The Montana Standard
Butte, Montana

KXLF-TV
Butte, Montana

Montana Television Network
Great Falls, Montana

Brooke Cadwallader
Economic Consultant
Dallas, Texas

Debbie Tyler
Publicist
Miami, Florida

Albert Rosenfeld
Consultant on Future Programs
National Foundation-March of Dimes
White Plains, New York

Dinah K. Lawrence
Typist
Butte, Montana

Allan Sonnenschein
Penthouse
New York, New York

Contents

Introduction

About 1200 Americans will die of cancer each day of this year—some 400,000 in all. These are our neighbors, our friends, our relatives.

Next year, adjusting for population growth, the rate of deaths from cancer will be two percent *higher*, and will increase at the same rate into the indefinite future. No wonder some have described this situation as a cancer "epidemic."

Since 1971, government expenditures on cancer have totaled more than *$5 billion.* In 1980–81, the U.S. government bill was $1 billion. The American Cancer Society (ACS) spent an additional $40 million on research.

And what are your chances of survival (five-year remission without clinical symptoms) if cancer strikes?

In the words of the American Cancer Society, your odds are "up to one in three." For some kinds of cancer, such as cancer of the esophagus, the odds are closer to one in twenty-five.

For comparison, let us turn to the past and Dr. Ellice McDonald of the Cancer Research Laboratories, Graduate School of Medicine, University of Pennsylvania, writing in the July 1931 issue of *Science*: "The very best we can hope for is to cure one-third of all cancer cases, obviously a confession of failure."

Ironically, if you had contracted cancer in 1931 and had found the right physicians, your odds would have surpassed those of 1981!

Is something wrong?

In this carefully documented book we hope to answer that question. We believe, contrary to official dogma, that incontrovertible evidence shows an association of bacteria with cancers of all kinds. We believe that a preventive vaccine is a practical and virtually immediate possibility. We believe that the course of "official" cancer research approaches one of the greatest scandals of all time. Further, we believe that nothing will be done about this unless the American people demand that something be done. For the first time we are going to tell the story of many years of important research on cancer—research that has been vilified, suppressed, and ignored.

In December 1979, on the basis of the manuscript version of this book, Senator John Melcher of Montana introduced a bill in the United States Senate to provide for research funding through the Department of Agriculture for part of the material we are going to describe (see Chapter 9).

Once you have read this book, we suggest that you write to your senators and representatives, demanding a full investigation.

On December 1, 1977, after author Netterberg presented them with the information, NBC

Nightly News presented to the nation the basic scientific facts indicating that the possibility for a universal cancer preventive vaccine does exist. A controlled study with the vaccine on animals was 70 percent effective in preventing the development of cancer, tested against five different tumor types. NBC News spent several months checking out the data before airing the presentation. What was the result of their exciting news report?

Three years of silence from the cancer establishment.

The Cancer Conspiracy

1

The Pioneers—Scott, Deaken, Glover

On Sunday morning, June 15, 1924, the *Anaconda* [Montana] *Standard* declared the good news in 54-point type:

DR. SCOTT TELLS OF CURE FOR DREAD CANCER PLAGUE[1]

Fifty-five years later, most of us reading this, secure in our belief that the answers to most problems lie in the scientists' hands, will scoff and whisper, "Quack!" For quite obviously the "dread cancer plague" is still very much with us.

But what if Scott was right?

Who was Scott and what had he discovered?

A 1903 graduate of Creighton University School of Medicine, Dr. Michael J. Scott came to Butte, Montana, then a thriving mining community at the height of its prosperity, in 1908. He became attached to St. James Hospital and eventually became its chief of staff.

Scott was a skilled surgeon and attracted patients from everywhere in the state. He did not think about alternatives to conventional cancer therapy—surgery and radiation treatment with radium needles—until he himself developed cancer in his left hand, a kind of "radiation-induced" cancer typically found in early users of X-rays. One of his close friends was the Reverend Charles B. Moulinier, S.J., president of the Catholic Hospital Association. Father Moulinier urged Scott to go to New York, where Moulinier had heard of a doctor who had developed a serum treatment for cancer. The doctor's name was Thomas J. Glover.[2]

Glover turned out to be a somewhat secretive, reticent man, for reasons we shall point out, but he did show Scott some animals with bacterially induced cancers and some slides of the stained bacillus—a bacterial microbe. Scott immediately recognized that if Glover was right about the bacterial connection with cancer, an antitoxin analogous to the antitoxin for diphtheria could be developed. Glover assured him that development of such an antitoxin was already in progress.

Scott made several more trips to New York, finally obtaining some of the serum, which was made by injecting horses with the killed bacterial microbe, then drawing out the serum from the blood, purifying and diluting it. He injected some of the serum into himself without ill effects. Since he was not yet sure of the efficacy of the serum, he decided that the second finger of his right hand had to be amputated. This was done by a surgeon friend in Portland, Oregon.

Scott's cancer did not spread, but since he had resorted to surgery, he could not prove to himself that the serum had prevented it from spreading.

Scott began to experiment with the so-called Glover cancer bacterium, running it through the famous test discovered by Robert Koch (1834–1910), a pioneer German bacteriologist. The experimenter using Koch's method injects the live bacterial microbe into an animal, causing the disease, then retrieves the same microbe from the tissues of the animal. Scott achieved positive results—as Glover had claimed. He decided to back Glover financially and began to borrow on valuable local property he owned in Montana.

According to his reports, Scott first used the serum on a 39-year-old woman with cancer of the breast.[3] This woman originally went to Rochester for surgery, with a letter of introduction from Scott to his friend, Charles Mayo. The woman's left breast was removed, along with the chest muscles and glands in the armpit. She was also given radiation treatment. Within a year, Scott found that the woman had new cancer in the right hand, arm, armpit, and collarbone. Further surgery was out of the question. The patient refused more radiation treatment. Scott began to administer the serum he had obtained from Glover. Within three months, the soreness and swelling began to leave the afflicted arm and hand. By January of 1923, she was apparently free of all evidence of cancer. The woman died at the age of 76, not from cancer but from injuries suffered in a fall.

Another case might further indicate the nature of Scott's success with his treatment. S. L., a woman of 53, had a diagnosed cancer of the pyloric end of the stomach. It was considered to be inoperable, and the patient was anemic, weak, losing weight, and practically bedridden. Scott began treatment in July of 1922, and the woman was able to resume her teaching duties again in the fall. In December, she reported that she was eating well and feeling no discomfort. She was still in good health in April 1924.

In addition to these two, ten other case histories were documented in the *Irish Journal of Cancer* in 1926.

In another report, in the April 1925 issue of *Northwest Medicine*, Scott optimistically saw promise in the bacteriological approach for a diagnostic blood test for cancer or even susceptibility to cancer. Indeed, he wrote:

> Results already obtained encourage us in the hope that it will be but a comparatively short time until carcinoma will be placed on the list of preventable diseases, prevention being accomplished through the establishment of an immunity to the carcinoma organism.[4]

In 1923, Scott left Butte for New York, where he could spend more time working with Glover and his laboratory assistant, Tom Deaken. Dr. Scott also managed to distribute serum to several physician friends and gave talks before many medical gatherings and associations.

As he worked with Glover, Scott discovered that the clever technical work on the bacillus was designed and carried out not by Glover, but by Deaken, a talented, self-educated man who had learned something about handling microbes in another laboratory and on his own had invented the rather elaborate culture medium necessary to grow the bacteria successfully outside the body. Independently, Deaken had carefully studied the bacterium extracted from cancerous tissue and described its unusual life cycle and its change of form, including one filterable form comparable to a virus. At the time, this was contrary to bacteriological theory, although the bacterium had been described by Dr. James Young of Edinburgh and others.[5]

Scott became an ardent apostle of "the parasitic origin of carcinoma" and traveled endlessly, soliciting support for this research and encouraging physicians to try the serum.

What happened to Scott is what has occurred again and again. Certainly no fool, no laboratory bungler, certainly no quack, since he lost his fortune in research, he had made what would seem to be the most logical assumption about cancer, because his therapy, based on that assumption, worked. Yet he was silenced.

If Scott had not developed cancer of the hand, would he himself have listened if another scientist had come forth with this bacterial theory? We should never underestimate the great inertia of institutionalized medicine or other sciences. Scott approached the influential leaders of the medical profession and was spurned, and soon the forces of orthodoxy began to freeze Scott out. For example, in 1926, at the invitation of Father Moulinier, he was scheduled to speak at a meeting of the Catholic Hospitals Association, but he was blocked from appearing on the regular program. Moulinier arranged for Scott to speak at a meeting after the official meeting closed, but powerful medical establishment forces were at work to stop him from appearing on the official program.

Scott eventually left New York for Butte, where he performed his last surgery about 1929. He then went to Seattle. He became a forgotten man—except to those "doomed" patients to whom he had given many years of life. A devout Catholic, Scott tried to find support for his work at Catholic colleges, seeking out some medical department that would continue his experiments. But orthodoxy prevailed, the medical world ironically having become as dogmatic as the Church had been in the days of Galileo.

Scott died in California in 1967, hopeful to the end. As far as official science was concerned, Scott had been dead a long time, but the issue was not closed. Indeed, if nothing more had come of it, the story of Scott would be the story of a Don Quixote, albeit with some puzzling cures.

In 1958, Dr. Robert E. Netterberg, one of the authors and a dentist in Butte, Montana, became interested in the cancer project when a Catholic priest, Father John F. McCarthy, told him of Dr. M. J. Scott's story. The priest had met Dr. Scott a few months previously, when Scott was visiting the Montana area. He had been living in Seattle and was almost eighty years old. In relating the story to Dr. Netterberg, the priest recounted what Dr. Scott had told him. He said that by the year 1924, in New York City, a common laboratory assistant and clean-up boy named Thomas J. Deaken had discovered a special culture medium for isolating and growing certain bacterial microbes from cancer tissue, blood, or urine from cancer patients or animals. Further tests had produced cancer in animals by injection of the microbes. Development of specific antiserum and vaccine against these bacterial microbes had produced astounding results in cancer patients.

Although very skeptical, at the urging of his friend, Dr. Netterberg decided to investigate the matter and brought Dr. Scott from Seattle to his own home, where he stayed for several weeks. Dr. Netterberg carefully went over Dr. Scott's published scientific papers, all of which had been published in reputable medical journals of the 1920s, and found them to be quite authentic. Proceeding from there, he contacted the major cancer research organizations in the United States, including the National Cancer Institute (NCI), and sent them the procedures that Dr. Scott had documented in 1924–26 showing the bacterial relation to cancer. He explained to Dr. Scott that surely this was just a matter of bringing the truth to the attention of the proper people. Dr. Netterberg felt certain that when these people discovered this apparently overlooked evidence, they would be quick to acknowledge the bacterial relation to cancer and would take immediate steps to assure the development of specific antisera and vaccines.

But Dr. Netterberg was rebuffed by all segments of the cancer establishment. In short, he was told that there was no evidence that cancer was infectious or that bacterial microbes had any connection with the disease. The "official" sources further claimed that previous studies in this area had proved that such bacterial microbes were mere contaminants. A pamphlet sent from the American Cancer Society stated emphatically that cancer is not caused by microbial infection.

Dr. Netterberg then proceeded to contact most of the major pharmaceutical manufacturing firms in the nation, in an attempt to interest them in developing the specific antiserum Dr. Scott had used in the 1920s. It was a waste of time. One company made a brief attempt at isolating the bacterial microbes but was unsuccessful. In the meantime, Dr. Netterberg spent many months tracking down two of the cancer patients that Dr. Scott had cured of advanced cancer and whose cases were written up in the *Irish Journal of Cancer* in 1926. After being declared terminally ill with cancer, both had lived into old age and were completely free of cancer decades later. They confirmed that Dr. Scott had been branded a cancer quack by his medical colleagues in the 1920s.

From complete skepticism, Dr. Netterberg was now convinced that there was much more to this story than met the eye. Why did he encounter such opposition when a few simple tests would indicate whether or not all of this was valid?

Digging further, Dr. Netterberg located other scientists who had confirmed the findings of Deaken and Scott about the bacterial microbe. Again the National Cancer Institute and the American Cancer Society were contacted. There was no interest.

In 1961, Dr. Netterberg took the entire story to Albert Rosenfeld, who was then science editor of *Life* magazine. After months of checking, the July 22, 1962, issue of *Life* was released, carrying headlines on the cover announcing new evidence that cancer may be infectious. Most of the story centered around virus research within various segments of the cancer establishment. A special page at the close of the story, set off from the main article, pictured two European scientists who had been confirming what Dr. Scott announced in 1924 about the bacterial microbes. The *Life* story aroused no interest or concern in the cancer powers about the idea that cancer might be a bacteria-related disease.

For the past twenty or more years, Dr. Netterberg has stayed with this project, digging and piecing together the fragments of evidence that cancer is somehow a bacteria-related disease. He has located other, contemporary scientists who hold high research positions and who have carried the bacterial discovery much further than Dr. Scott did. These scientists have testified before the United States Congress that they cannot receive funding for research that may lead to the development of a universal cancer vaccine through the use of certain bacterial microbes. Dr. Netterberg has contacted many members of the press to make them aware of the history of this long-suppressed discovery and the current scientific results that are proving that the original 1924 announcements were valid.

2

What Is Cancer?

In order to understand what cancer is, we must first examine the structure and function of normal cells. A cell—the basic unit of all life, plant or animal—is composed of protoplasm surrounded by the cell membrane. Inside the protoplasm is a round body called the nucleus, which contains the chromosomes and genes. In each species of mammals the number of chromosomes differs. In human beings, they number 46. The nucleus is surrounded by its own membrane within the cell. The nuclei of bacteria, however, do not have a membrane.

The nucleus of a human cell functions like a computer, as the genes govern the physiology of the cell and its dividing processes to form new cells. This "computer" mechanism allows the cell to breathe, process food for survival, excrete wastes, and synthesize enzymes, hormones, or other substances.

One-celled creatures, such as bacteria, often do everything necessary for life support and reproduction. In complex creatures, however, the cells specialize during fetal development, according to instructions programmed in the genetic code. Genes also determine hereditary characteristics in the individual. Each gene acts as a center of specific chemical activity.

A most interesting metaphor has been devised by Arthur Koestler to describe this phenomenon:

> Let the chromosomes be represented by the keyboard of a grand piano—a very grand piano with thousands of keys. Then each key will be a gene. Every cell in the body carries a microscopic but complete keyboard in its nucleus. But each specialized cell is only permitted to sound one chord, according to its specialty—the rest of its genetic keyboard has been inactivated by Scotch tape. The fertilized egg, and the first few generations of its daughter cells, had the complete keyboard at their disposal. But successive generations have, at each "point of no return" larger and larger areas of it covered by Scotch tape. In the end, a muscle cell can only do one thing: contract—strike a single chord.
>
> The Scotch tape is known in the language of genetics as the "repressor." The agent which strikes a key and activates the gene is an "inducer." A mutated gene is a key which has gone out of tune.[1]

In healthy people the cells do their jobs, repair damage when it occurs, and exist in an incredibly harmonious equilibrium.

Under the microscope, a normal cell has clear features. The cytoplasm that surrounds the nucleus is transparent, and the nucleus is well defined within the cell. The cell is literally the picture of health.

But many things can go wrong in a cellular

mechanism, from wounds to poisoning of the cell by chemicals, radiation, or infection. One such malfunction is what we could call "malignant transformation," the *uncontrolled* reproduction of a cell. According to current theory, such malignant transformations take place in each one of us from birth, but our *immune system* recognizes the transformed cell as defective and repairs or kills it. The reason for these continual transformations is the instability of DNA, the chemical carrier of heredity.

Then sometime in life, a transformed cell may mature and get a head start on the immune system—a process we shall describe in greater detail later in this book—and then we have what is called *cancer*, the clinical term for a process always taking place, *but now out of control.*

Under the microscope, the nucleus of a cancer cell appears irregular in shape and sometimes larger than the nucleus of a healthy cell. The nucleus looks clumped together and may, in fact, subdivide into multiple nuclei. The whole cell takes on an irregular appearance. Some type of chemical change has obviously occurred within the nucleus of the cell to cause this transformation.

The dividing cancer cells form a mass that is voracious in its demand for blood and nutriments. Unlike benign (nonmalignant) tumors, which are contained in a "capsule," malignant tumors are large and irregular in shape and disordered in their spatial pattern.

The main characteristic of the cancer cell, which makes it so life-threatening, is its ability to invade surrounding normal tissue. Cells can also separate from the malignant tumor and travel to other parts of the body, where they seem able to "infect" new sites. Unaffected by the usual immunal barriers in the body, these invading cells become new lumps of cancer. Cancer cells may also spread by way of the lymphatic systems and the blood. This spreading is called *metastasis*. Invasion and metastasis are the two fundamental characteristics of malignancy.

Cancer cells have been described as primitive or "embryonic," a concept of importance, as we shall later show.

Some cancers divide and spread very quickly—for example, melanoma, a malignancy of pigment cells that make up natural brownish spots in the skin. Other cancers are slow. An example of a slow-growing cancer is cancer of the prostate. It is like a turtle; its invasion is slow but sure.

Cancer is diagnosed primarily by two methods—biopsy (histopathology) and smear (cytology). In the biopsy, a small piece of suspected tissue is sectioned and stained by the pathologist and examined under the microscope. He looks for the changes in cellular characteristics that we have just described. In some cases, if the cellular transformation has not reached a discernible stage, it may be difficult for him to diagnose accurately whether or not the cells are truly malignant. If the changes are significant, there will be no problem determining that they are cancer cells. In cytology, cells per se, obtained from a smear or where they can be aspirated, as from the lung, are examined under the microscope. The well known Papanicolaou (Pap) smear is a cytological method of determining the presence of cancer cells, although it is limited primarily to the detection of cancer cells of the cervix. The Pap smear is based upon the principle that cancer cells can be identified through the use of special staining techniques. Here again, the cytologist looks for physical, visible changes in cells.

As for early diagnosis of cancer, biopsy and the Pap smear have been the only major advancements. The tools that the pathologist must use are relatively crude. The biopsy test has not changed in fifty years. Although there have been some improvements in staining techniques, both biopsy and smear methods have reached the limits of their development. It is unlikely that they can be improved. The question is now, and has always been, how early can chemical changes be detected in the cell before it becomes a cancer cell? Until now, no reliable chemical test has been developed. Consequently, the pathologist must rely on visual techniques using the microscope.

It has long been known that cancer cells have the ability to synthesize various chemical compounds. However, until recently, efforts to pinpoint one chemical factor for *all* cancer cells have failed. Perhaps this failure has contributed to the belief that there are many forms of cancer, all differing from each other. Should a chemical substance be found that is being synthesized uniquely by every cell classified as a cancer cell, that would constitute a long-sought-after common denominator and permit, for the first time, the definition of what a cancer cell actually is. Such a discovery would also present a possible method for early detection of cancer, through a test for the presence and concentration of this common chemical. That common denominator has been found, as we shall detail in another chapter.

As we have said, cancer is probably always present is us. A few cells are constantly beginning to acquire malignant characteristics, but our immune system keeps them under control. The number of cells undergoing transformation in a one-year-old child, however, is much fewer than the number of such cells in a twenty-year-old. This is because the twenty-year-old has been subjected to a lengthier attack from irritants, be they his own bodily products; carcinogens in the air, food, and water; or natural and man-made radiation.

A forty-year-old individual has suffered even more exposure to these factors. The longer the exposure to these elements, the greater the risk that cells will become malignant. This risk is further enhanced by many other factors. Even if a person were isolated from the known environmental causes of cancer, he would not be entirely safe because he would be exposed to his own body products. If immunological resistance is reduced, cancer cells can develop and survive to continue their multiplication and destruction. This is undoubtedly why only 5 to 8 percent of cancer cases occur in children, since children have not had this exposure to these carcinogenic elements.

The causes of cancer have long been in dispute. Most theories were stated by 1925, when Scott listed them: (a) embryonic rests—cells left over or arrested in embryonic development; (b) injury, inflammation, and chronic irritation; (c) chemical irritants; (d) metabolism disturbances; (e) changes in internal secretions; (f) senile changes; and (g) bacterial infection. The official favorites at the present time are the carcinogens—chemical elements or compounds, many of which can cause cell mutations—and the viruses.

3

Treating and Preventing Cancer

Once cancer has been diagnosed by the methods described, treatment begins.

Historically, surgery was the first effective approach to cancer, and such is the case today, except for a few types, such as cancer of the prostate, which seem to respond better to other treatment. A large cancer mass is a formidable target, however, and even if destroyed by the other kinds of treatment, it can be toxic in its decomposition. Surgery has become more sophisticated in the twentieth century, although certain surgical procedures are still controversial, such as radical mastectomy for breast cancer or prophylactic removal of breasts from teenage girls with a family history of cancer.

Since the time of Becquerel and the Curies, radiation has been the second line of attack on cancer cells. The use of radiation has always been paradoxical, since everyone in the atomic age knows that radiation can *cause* cell damage and, eventually, cancer. However, early success against certain kinds of cancer by the use of radium needles (hollow needles filled with radium or radon gas) made it standard treatment for many cancers, up to the end of World War II.

Present-day radiation technology uses high-intensity gamma-radiation from radioactive cobalt. Radiation damages and destroys rapidly dividing cells, and since cancer cells often grow more rapidly than most normal cells, the cancer cells are damaged the most. Also, of course, the radiation can be focused. Side effects of radiation are the suppression of the immune system and damage of normal tissue.

Although attempts to find substances that would halt the growth of external cancers go back as far as surgery, chemotherapy has its scientific roots in the technology of modern warfare. Mustard gas, a highly poisonous gas used in World War I, can burn the skin, the lining of the lungs, and the intestines with agonizing and frequently fatal results. An accident with mustard gas in World War II (when it was *not* used in combat) exposed a number of people to nonfatal amounts of the substance. Survivors showed a sharp decrease in white blood cells. This suggested that some form of mustard gas might be useful against leukemia, a cancer involving the tissues that form white blood cells.

The search for chemical agents that will attack cancer without killing the patient outright has been a major thrust of modern cancer research. So far, a number of cancer-fighting chemicals have been developed and discovered. One group, known as the alkylating agents, is related chemically to mustard gas. These chemical agents affect

DNA and disturb cell division. They have toxic effects on bone marrow and often cause the baldness characteristic of patients being treated by chemotherapy.

Another group, known technically as the antimetabolites, either substitute for some vital chemical used by cancer cells or block the formation of nucleic acid.

A number of toxic antibiotics, such as Actinomycin, derived from bacteria and fungi, have some uses. All are extremely poisonous.

Other drugs have specific effects on cancer cell growth and metabolism. The use of Laetrile would probably count as chemotherapy, since in theory the active substance should release hydrocyanic acid at the site of cancer cells but not at the sites of normal cells.

Virtually all of the various chemicals used in cancer therapy have side effects, many of them so severe that some authorities have stated that if the patient can survive the chemotherapy, he might also survive the cancer. Undesirable effects range from simple nausea to bone marrow and intestinal damage.

Since at least one theory of cancer suggests that the healthy immune system keeps malignant transformations of cells from becoming clinically cancerous, failure of the immune system because of age, illness, heredity, sedentary life, or even emotional stress may be a major factor in cancer. For many scientists, immunology seems to be the most promising area of future therapy.[1]

One of the mavericks of cancer research, whose treatments were long on the American Cancer Society's list of "unproven therapies," was Dr. William B. Coley, who at the end of the nineteenth century infected cancer patients with erysipelas, a bacterial disease characterized by high fever. His patients frequently showed improvement or actual remission of the cancers. Immunologists have found Coley's work of interest, and agents such as tuberculosis bacteria (BCG) have been used to stimulate the immune system of cancer patients. Recent animal studies have suggested that other chemicals (one example being synthetic muramyl dipeptides and trehalose dimycolate) can stimulate the immune system to attack cancers without some of the difficulties involved in using live bacteria.[2]

Unfortunately, immunological treatment of cancer is not widespread.

One of the incredible and disquieting facts about cancer therapy taken as a whole is the lack of agreement among experts. For example, when the *New England Journal of Medicine*, perhaps the most prestigious of medical journals, publishes an authoritative report on a cancer treatment, the following issues will contain letters from other experts who have information on some other technique that they think is better. In the words of Alexander Pope, "Who shall decide when doctors disagree?"

In the prevention of cancer, surprisingly little has been learned, but prevention on the whole has not been a major target of research. The search for carcinogens—substances that damage cells and ultimately cause cancer—was undoubtedly intended as a step toward preventing cancer, but the vast number of such substances in the factory, the school, the home, the air, the food, and the water has created a dismal picture indeed. Even if one does not work in an asbestos plant or live under the smokestack of a chemical factory, one still has to breathe, drink, and eat, and continual exposure to carcinogens is a fact of life for everyone, although in varying intensities.

Jean McCann published articles in the *Medical Tribune* (November 22, 1978) and in *Good Housekeeping* (May 1979) summarizing the opinions of twelve experts on cancer prevention. The group included Dr. Benjamin Bird, Jr., professor of clinical surgery, Vanderbilt University School of Medicine and a past president of the American Cancer Society; Dr. Arthur Holleb, director of medical affairs, American Cancer Society; Dr. John H. Knowles, president of the Rockefeller Foundation; Dr. Linus Pauling, head of the Linus Pauling Institute of Medicine and Society; Dr. Fred Rapp, chairman of the Department of Microbiology and director of the Specialized Cancer Research Center, Pennsylvania State University College of Medicine, Hershey, Pennsylvania; Dr. Avery A. Sandberg, chief, Department of Medicine, Roswell Park Memorial Institute, Buffalo, New York; Dr. Thomas Slaga head of skin carcinogenesis and tumor-prevention group, Oak Ridge National Laboratory, Oak Ridge, Tennessee; Dr. Arthur Upton, former director of the National Cancer Institute; Dr. Elizabeth Whalen, research associate at the Harvard School of Public Health; Dr. Roger Williams, biochemist, University of Texas; Dr. Warren Winkelman, Jr., dean and professor of epidemiology, University of California, Berkeley; and Dr. Ernest L. Wynder, president of the American Health Foundation.

Among the things the group suggested we avoid are the following (number of responses in parentheses):

Smoking (5)
High-fat diets (4)
Food additives (2)
Sunbathing (1)
Sugar (1)
Radiation (1)

Positive recommendations included the following:

Vitamin C in doses from minimum daily requirement to 10 grams (5)
Other vitamins, such as A and E (4)
Exercise (3)
High-fiber diet (3)
Weight control (2)
Mammography for women over 50 (2)
Flavones in vegetables such as cauliflower (1)

Most of these suggestions come from evidence uncovered by various researchers. One such discovery was that nitrites found in bacon and other preserved meat form a carcinogenic chemical in the body, the formation of which can be prevented by Vitamin C.

While a person following all of the dos and

don'ts will probably be healthy and less likely to get cancer, the lack of agreement is disquieting, considering the vast cost of cancer research in the past decade.

4

The Persistent Quest

We have already noted that Dr. Scott learned about the cancer antiserum from Thomas Glover and his assistant, Tom Deaken. After Scott had retreated to poverty and obscurity, Glover and his associates continued with important work on cancer.

In 1940, Dr. Glover and Dr. John E. White, a surgeon from Malone, New York, published a report titled *The Treatment of Cancer in Man: Results Obtained in the Treatment of Cancer in Man with a Specific Antiserum.*[10]

In the beginning of the work, the authors describe the preparation of the antiserum as we have discussed in a previous chapter. They also point out that surgery was often necessary, along with administering specific cancer antiserum, because of the massive bulk of the tumors involved.

This report deals with the successful treatment of 328 patients from the early 1920s to 1939. The cases include, in order, tumors of the scalp, face, nose, lip, mouth, tongue, neck, breast, arm, hand, prepuce (foreskin of the penis), perineum, anus, and foot, then gastrointestinal tumors, and finally tumors of the female reproductive organs.

The report covers literally hundreds of patients, with both operable and inoperable cancer, who had been free of the disease up to twelve years since treatment, and all of whom were within the five-year remission period considered "cure" by the contemporary cancer establishment.

In *The Treatment of Cancer in Man*, Glover and White also tell that in 1929, Dr. George McCoy, director of the Hygienic Laboratory (later named the National Institutes of Health), visited Glover's New York laboratory at the Murdock Foundation to observe the work being done in the study of cancer-related bacteria and in antiserum therapy. McCoy then invited Glover and his associates to repeat *under supervision* their experiments with the bacteria.

The group included, besides Glover and White, Dr. George A. Clark, a pathologist at Scranton, Pennsylvania; and Dr. J. L. Engle.

The work began in December 1929, and continued until the summer of 1938. Not all the workers were in Washington during this entire period, however.

In March of 1933, Dr. McCoy authorized the publication of a paper describing the production of a malignant adenoma (gland) in the breast of a guinea pig by inoculation with a bacteria cultured from human cancer tissue. Only one case was chosen, to soften what McCoy rightly estimated as a "salvo" of adverse criticism. Opposition to their work and the theory of the bacterial cause of cancer did lead to the marshaling of greater opposition in 1937 and 1938.

By 1937, a thorough study of the bacteria had been made at the laboratories, and the workers pressed for publication of a report on their work. McCoy agreed.

Before publication could be arranged, however, McCoy was replaced as head of the laboratory by Dr. R. H. Thompson, who appointed a special committee of five members of the National Institutes of Health (NIH). This committee recommended the publication of three papers: one on the bacteriology, one on the work with guinea pigs, and one on the work with rats. On the recommendation of three members of the committee, the paper on the guinea pig work was to be done first.

When this paper had been prepared, the committee suggested some revision but again recommended publication by the Public Health Service.

Meanwhile, the surgeon general decided that a member of the National Advisory Cancer Council should sit with the committee. After discussion, the majority again voted to publish.

Then the assistant surgeon general and the director of the NIH suggested that a footnote be appended to the paper, relieving the NIH of any responsibility of concurring with the findings, although the work had been done in *their* laboratories! As Glover writes: "It is to be noted that this suggestion was made notwithstanding the fact that at the commencement of the work, a request had been made by the authors that there should be constant supervision of their work by one or more competent members of the Staff."[10]

A memorandum from McCoy to the assistant surgeon general stated that McCoy still regarded the work as perhaps the most important work on cancer done during his supervision of the laboratory.

In place of the desired footnote taking the NIH off the hook, the authors pointed out in the introduction to the report that they had asked for supervision but had not usually received it because of lack of qualified personnel. The paper was then submitted to the committee, which once again voted *for* publication!

Surgeon General Parran then instructed McCoy to write a foreword. McCoy complied, with a short preface backing the work, although somewhat cautiously. Then at a conference attended by the surgeon general, director Thompson, and two minority members of the committee, it was moved that the work be repeated by one of the staff of the NIH before publication.

Since eight years of work had gone into the animal studies, since repetition of the work would take at least two more years, and since publication would still not be assured, the authors decided to publish their results privately. It is obvious, even at this distance, that every attempt was made to suppress this historical confirmation of the bacterial relationship to cancer that Dr. M. J. Scott had announced in detail in 1924. When in 1977 author Netterberg tried to get copies of the NIH records directly from the NIH, he was told that they were lost!

Fortunately, however, for posterity and history, the researchers had preserved copies of the official serial-numbered records of the confirmation, dating back to 1935. Consequently, in 1938, Glover and Engle published a booklet titled *Studies in Malignancy: Production of Metastasizing Tumors in Guinea Pigs and Albino Rats Following the Innoculation of a Bacterial Suspension Containing a Micro-Organism Obtained from Human Cancer.*[9]

In 1953, another member of the group, Dr. George A. Clark, presented a report on the same work at the Third International Conference on Microbiology at Rome, Italy.[4] At this scientific meeting Dr. Clark tried to make known the results that had been solidly verified eighteen years before! In his report, Dr. Clark describes how they were suppressed.

What had Dr. Clark and his associates accomplished within the NIH by 1935? Let us examine these findings.

1. They had taken thirty-seven specimens of malignant tissue from humans and animals and made bacterial cultures from them. Many "types" of cancer were tested, and all of the culture work was done under the strictest sterile conditions to rule out contamination by outside bacteria, which might have entered the cultures. In *every* case, the tissue culture tested positive for "Glover's organism," which they describe as a pleomorphic bacterium—that is, one that changes form with different conditions of temperature, dryness, culture medium, and maturity, sometimes being a rod, a sphere, a chain of spheres, and a filterable spore

form. Other well-known bacteria that exhibit similar behavior are the bacteria of tuberculosis and leprosy.

2. They managed to adapt the bacteria isolated from human cancerous tissue to guinea pigs, then to rats, then back to guinea pigs again, until both the rats and guinea pigs developed malignant tumors. Meticulous adaptation charts were kept of the passage from animal to animal in order to document its "take" ability, since it was originally a bacterial strain from a human breast carcinoma. The malignant tumors that developed were all biopsied, photographed, and verified by pathologists. All records were numbered under official Hygienic Laboratory and NIH rules.

The authors have had these detailed serial-numbered NIH records reviewed by expert scientists. The scientists have given their professional opinion that the confirmation work on the bacterial microbes of cancer was done well, absolutely fulfilling Koch's postulates that the microbes are involved in the causation of cancer. The pains taken, for example, to insure sterility of the culture media, would do justice to a modern laboratory. Here was another major turning point for the conquest of cancer—confirmed proof of what Dr. M. J. Scott had announced by 1924. But it was again stifled by the official powers, who could see no further than to make charges of "contamination" when bacteria were isolated from cancer patients.

A separate report by Dr. White in 1953 at the same congress in Rome,[25] shows the general effectiveness of this treatment. His cures within a group of 100 patients averaged 54 percent, a considerably better average than present-day statistics. His cures ranged from 100 percent in the case of colon and bone cancers to 10 percent on prostate cancer and 0 percent on tongue and liver cancer.

In one of Dr. White's typical cases, an eight-year-old girl was brought to him in May 1928. She had previously been treated for a cystic tumor of the right antrum (part of the nasal passage). When she came to White, he reported: "This girl is pale and poorly nourished. She complains of a constant pain in the region of the right antrum. The right upper lip and cheek are swollen and edematous [excessive accumulation of fluid]. In the mouth, on the buccal surface of the gum, above the site of the right upper second molar tooth is a red fibril mass about one inch by one-half inch in area."

White began serum treatment and removed the mass in the mouth by endothermy (electric scalpel). The pathology report was "osteogenic sarcoma," cancer arising from the bone. White continued serum treatment until July 1929, at which time "all evidence of the disease disappeared. In August 1950, the patient, then thirty years of age and the mother of two healthy-appearing children, came to call. A note in 1951 tells us that she is fine."

At about the same time, W. M. Crofton, M.D., Lecturer in Special Pathology at University College, Dublin, Ireland, published a heretical book titled *The True Nature of Viruses.*[5] Crofton claimed to have isolated so-called viruses from victims of several diseases and to have succeeded in growing a "streptothrix" (a bacterial microbe) from each. He said that a microbe was always associated with cancer, a bacterium pleomorphic in character, or perhaps more than one microbe. He also made vaccines from the bacterial forms, which he used with surprising success. Crofton described the mechanism of cancer thus:

> In cancer, the fertilization of the cell-nucleus is produced by the virus phase of the microbe—of a streptothrix in sarcoma—of commonly a staphylococcus in carcinoma—and it is the cell invaded by the particular microbe and the nature of the microbe that determines the particular form of tumor. The virus has the same effect on the nucleus it invades as the head of a spermatozoon, changing the nature of the cell from a peaceful citizen contributing to the welfare of the community into one whose ferments enable it to prey on its fellows. [5]

Crofton's work was bitterly attacked, and he found it impossible to publish articles, although others confirmed his techniques and results. He had private booklets printed, showing microphotographs of the microbes, trying to convince his peers that cancer is a bacteria-related disease, but he was ignored.

One prominent researcher who has dominated the field of cancer microbiology has been Dr. Virginia (Wuerthele-Caspe Livingston) Wheeler. A graduate of Vassar College, she received her M.D. degree from New York University. Her professional posts have included an associate professorship in research at Rutgers University, directorship of the Laboratory of Proliferative Disease at Presbyterian Hospital in Newark, New Jersey, and a research associateship at the San Diego Biomedical Institute. She is the founder and moving spirit of the Livingston-Wheeler Medical Clinic in San Diego, California. She has been outstandingly successful in cancer therapy through a combination of autogenous (from the patient) vaccines, diet, vitamins, and more conventional treatments.

In her book *Cancer: A New Breakthrough*, Dr. Livingston-Wheeler summarizes her view of cancer as follows:

> It is a natural state for all living things to be parasitized by various microbes, some helpful, some harmless, and some downright harmful. The harmful ones usually arouse a state of resistance in the host by means of various mechanisms such as antibodies, circulating and fixed white cells, enzymes and numerous other intricate biological processes that seek to restore the body to health. Sometimes the harmful microbes produce substances which prevent the host from reacting by elaboration of toxic materials or by masquerading as a harmless constituent of the body. Such an invader is the Hidden Killer, the *Progenitor Cryptocides*. It can exist in the human host as an ongoing, underlying chronic infection which, in the beginning, may be silent, but in the end, fulminates into an overpowering enemy.[16]

Dr. Wheeler began her study of bacteria-related disease in 1941, with an initial contact with scleroderma, a systemic and often fatal disease that begins with a hardening of the skin, often producing painful ulcers. A nurse friend had the disease and was seeking help. In 1946, Dr. Wheeler, Dr. Camille Mermon, a pathologist, and Dr. Eva Brodkin, a dermatologist, isolated (from two scleroderma patients) a bacterial organism similar to that of leprosy. They reported that cultures of the organism from human tissues caused sclerodermlike reactions in guinea pigs.[19] This discovery was later confirmed and published in scientific papers by Demotte and der Meiren in 1953[6] and by Cantwell and Kelso in 1971.[3]

This initial observation prompted the idea that cancer also might be caused by a bacterial microbe. By 1947, Dr. Wheeler was convinced that a bacterial microbe was in fact involved in the development of cancer, and that the microbe was probably of the family of microbes of tuberculosis and leprosy known as the *Actinomycetales* group. A colleague, Dr. Eleanor Alexander-Jackson, developed a special triple-staining process that, it was claimed, allowed them to distinguish the microbe from others of similar nature under the microscope.[1] Like Clark and others, she also described the microbe as being pleomorphic, having at various times under different conditions the form of rods, globes, spores, and a Seitz-filterable stage, whose size is comparable to that of a virus and which cannot be seen under the ordinary microscope. Virus-size microbes must be viewed under the electron microscope, which enlarges them many thousands of times. In other words, this microbe could be a bacterium but also enter a stage so small that it could not be detected by the standard microscope techniques for viewing bacteria.

In a paper in which Dr. Wheeler and her colleagues discuss their reasons for believing in the importance of this bacterium and its role in cancer,[15] Dr. James Hillier, an expert in electron microscopy, states categorically that a "microorganism is present and can be demonstrated with the proper technique in every type of human tumor and in animal tumors we have studied," including those caused by injection of fuel oil, a classic carcinogen.

An important paper in 1950 by Dr. Wheeler with Drs. Eleanor Alexander-Jackson, John A. Anderson, James Hillier, Roy Allen, and Lawrence D. Smith,[17] makes the important point that some pathogenic organisms (microbes that produce disease) are not species specific but can directly affect other hosts. Thus, even a virus thought to be specific to chickens in Rous Chicken Sarcoma, has been transmitted to mice and other laboratory animals. A report to the Rome conference of 1953[20] stressed this point and indicated that the microbe had passed Koch's test by producing cancer in animals that had been injected with it, as described earlier in this work.

A paper in 1953 with Dr. Eleanor Alexander-Jackson[23] relates the bacterial theory to the virus theory of such workers as Milford and Duran-Reynals, except that Wheeler and Jackson believe that the true causative agent is the filterable or viruslike stage of the bacterium rather than a true virus.

In 1956, Dr. Wheeler isolated from victims of Wilson's disease, a degenerative disease attacking the liver, a bacterial microbe similar to the one she felt was invariably associated with cancer.[19] Although larger than the cancer-related microbe, it had many of the same characteristics of pleomorphism, that is, the ability to change shape.

In 1965, a paper by Dr. Wheeler and Dr. Alexander-Jackson[15] reports that the chemical actinomycin was found in the urine and in cultures from cancer patients. The significance is that the most likely sources of this toxic chemical compound were bacteria from the *Actinomycetales* group. Actinomycin also has harmful effects upon the hormone balance of the body. It is important to point out these findings so that it can be seen to what painstaking tests these researchers subjected the microbes in order to properly classify them.

The finding of actinomycin led in turn to the proposition that the cancer-related bacterium could be classified as a member of the *Actinomycetales* group, a close cousin to the causative microbes of tuberculosis and leprosy. In Dr. Wheeler's opinion, this microbe was perhaps a primitive form of a number of harmful bacteria. She and Dr. Alexander-Jackson proposed the name of *Progenitor cryptocides* (ancestral hidden killer)[24] for this bacterium.

Among the characteristics used in classifying the microbe, she lists:

1. It can be classified as a virus.

2. It is acid-fast in some stages of its life cycle, meaning that it will retain the acid of a special type of staining procedure used on bacteria,

whereas, normally this stain would not be retained.

3. It lives in the intestinal tract of man.

4. It is in the red blood cells of the cancer patient and does not create a fever like some other disease-producing microbes do. It must be seen under the dark field microscope, like the causative microbe of syphilis.

A 1970 paper by Dr. Wheeler and several colleagues[11] discusses the discovery of other products besides actinomycin, although the nature of some of these was as yet unknown. In 1972, Dr. Wheeler described new, improved techniques for observing the microbe in the blood.

Meanwhile, in Europe other investigators were also isolating and observing the same organism and describing the exact same change-of-form life cycle. In each case, the same microbe was isolated from cancer patients. The Italian scientist Dr. Clara Fonti, for example, in a book published in 1958,[7] describes an experiment in which she injected herself in the chest wall with fluid from a metastasizing human breast cancer. After a few days an eruption appeared and finally a nut-sized lesion in the left breast. Biopsy examinations diagnosed the lesion as "baso-cellular epithelioma" (a form of cancer). After a period of several months, the lesions regressed. She made a serum that was specific to the bacterial microbes involved and cured herself. Then, she used the serum from her own blood, which presumably contained antibodies against these bacterial microbes of cancer, on a patient with multiple abdominal cancers. This resulted in improvement when the serum was injected over a period of time.

A German scientist, Franz Gerlach, in a book published in 1948,[8] describes prolonged observations of microorganisms cultured from thousands of samples of tumor tissue, blood, and other fluids of cancer patients. He describes the main bacterial microbe as a kind of micro-fungus, but his definitive description is very similar to that of the pleomorphic bacterium described by Dr. Wheeler and colleagues from 1941 to 1976 and by Dr. M. J. Scott in his announcements in the 1920s.

A 1973 paper by Florence Siebert, J. Kerking, and R. L. Davis of the Veterans Administration Center, Bay Pines, Florida,[14] reports on twenty-nine bacteria of various kinds isolated from human and rat tumors. *All* appeared to be pleomorphic.

Thus far we have seen that a number of researchers in various countries and at various times have described a microbe (or possibly microbes) cultured from cancer tissues—microbes that in turn could produce pathological conditions in test animals. In medicine and research the assigning of "cause" is a difficult problem, however, compounded by the fact that an ethical medical researcher cannot experiment on human beings if the experimentation is likely to be harmful or possibly fatal.

In view of the many studies we have reviewed, we are convinced that bacteria are associated in some way with cancer. We are less certain than some excellent scientists cited in this chapter that the relationship is casual. As our next chapter shall discuss, however, such a decision is not essential for the next step in defeating cancer.

The problem of the role of cancer-related microbes will be resolved in time, since paradoxes (microbe–no-microbe, etc.) rarely exist in nature, and the truth will eventually be realized.

In fact, we are convinced that in fifty years or less, with cancer gone the way of smallpox and tuberculosis, and with the realization that the scientists in the early 1920s were right about what cancer is, people will say of those who control cancer research, "How could they possibly not have known?"

5

The Fatal Embryonic Hormone

If the persistent scientists we have discussed in previous chapters had not sacrificed time, money, recognition, and even reputation to work on the problem of cancer-related bacteria, we doubt that the promising discoveries we are about to describe would have been made in our lifetime or, if made, understood. If, as we believe, the discoveries are among the most important in the history of biological science as well as in cancer research, then the work of these scientists will not have been in vain. Their faith in their work ultimately will be vindicated.

To understand these discoveries, we must again enter the world of normal cells and normal growth.

When egg and sperm unite in mammals, the original cell begins to divide, and the new creature, which is to become a human being or an animal, attaches itself to the wall of the uterus by layers of cells known technically as the trophoblast (literally "nourishing growth").

These cells synthesize and secrete a substance

with the jaw-breaking name *chorionic gonadotropin* or *choriogonadotropin*, which we will henceforth abbreviate CG. According to evidence now available,[14 34 37 39 40] one of the functions of CG is to protect the embryo, which, because it has chromosomes from the father, would be subject to attack as foreign matter. In 1976, this substance was also located in human spermatozoa.[1 6]

Since 1970, different investigators have also found the presence of a CG-like substance in the serum of a great number of patients with cancer,[9 10 34] suggesting that the cancer cells, like the trophoblasts and sperm, are also producers of CG or a CG-like substance. Further studies by investigators at Denver and Pittsburgh[2 41] demonstrated that cancer cells, irrespective of origin, type of cancer, and even *species*, do indeed synthesize the CG-like compound. These discoveries vindicate, in a sense, the pioneer scientist, Beard,[8] who in 1902 theorized that cancer cells were much like trophoblastic cells.

A most important scientific paper by Canadian researchers Malkin, Kellen, Cameron, and Farber, recently published in the *Scandinavian Journal of Immunology*,[30] reports that CG is present in *premalignant* liver cells in rats, suggesting that the production of CG is part of a "programmed phenomenon," again indicating that genes or DNA coding is involved and that the CG synthesis is actually part of the very physiology and development of the cancer cell.

The mechanism by which CG, on the surface of fetal cells, spermatozoa, and cancer cells, defends such cells, appears to be physico-chemical in nature. CG, because of the presence in its molecules of a substance called sialic acid, has a high-density negative electric charge.[24 35 43 45] Agents of the immune system also carry a negative electric charge, but of lesser magnitude. It is a basic principle of electricity that objects with similar electric charges repel each other, an effect easily demonstrated by the action of small, electrically charged foam balls or the leaves of a potentiometer.

Indeed, such agents of the immune system as the white blood cell macrophages cannot get close enough to attack the cancer cell, although the lymphocytes have signaled that the tissue is foreign. If, for example, you had a staph infection in your finger, the macrophages and lymphocytes would immediately go into action against the intruder. In the case of cancer, however, some of the immune system white blood cells become coated with CG themselves, and this renders them ineffective against the cells, even if they actually touch them.[7] The presence of CG in the cell membrane that surrounds the cancer cell, in quantities large enough to repeal the agents of the immune system, is a practical definition of malignant transformation or what we call cancer. (see Figures 1, 2, and 3.)

We have already discussed the work of Dr. Virginia Livingston-Wheeler in classifying and studying a microbe she has named *Progenitor cryptocides*. In a 1974 issue of *Transactions of the New York Academy of Sciences*,[44] Dr. Livingston-Wheeler announced a major medical research

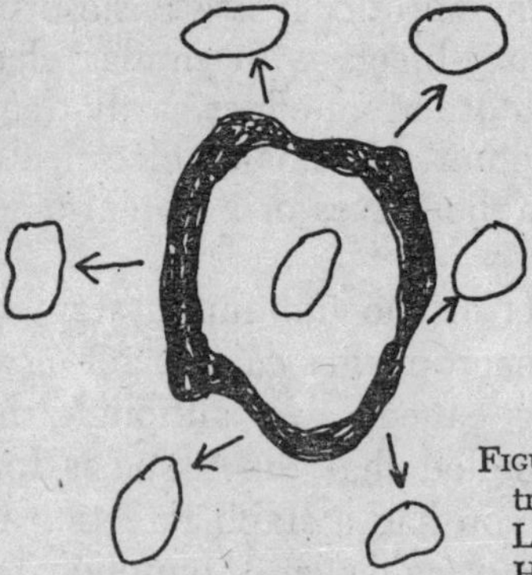

The CG-like hormone (black border) localizes in the outer membrane of the cancer cell, and its high negative electric charge wards off white blood cells preventing them from approaching and destroying the cell.

FIGURE 1. A Diagrammatic Illustration of Cancer Cell and the Localization of the CG-like Hormone in the Outer Membrane Wall.

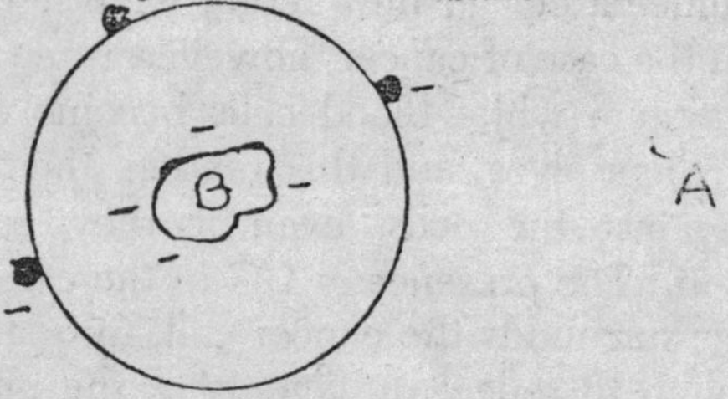

FIGURE 2. This represents a classic experiment. Foreign liver cells (A) were immediately attacked and devoured by agents of the immune system (black bodies). The cancer cell (B) is not attacked because the negative charges repel the agents of the immune system at a distance too far for destructive effects to reach the cell.

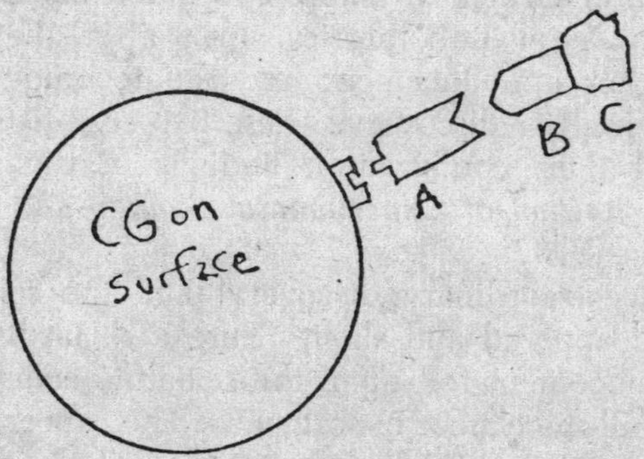

FIGURE 3. Antibody and double antibody action. The antibody A specifically will lock onto CG. Antibody B (from another animal) is specific to the A antibody and may carry a marker (C) such as radioactive iodine.

breakthrough: her own discovery and confirmation that the microbe of cancer also synthesizes a CG-like material much like the material synthesized by cancer cells. Her observation was confirmed by two other scientists, Drs. Herman Cohen and Alice Strampp, two noted biochemists of Princeton Laboratories, Inc., after they had read her announcement and the techniques for verifying her discovery. These two scientists published their confirmation findings in the prestigious *Journal of Experimental Biology and Medicine* in 1976.[13]

An extraordinary discovery! Did the scientific world applaud and shout "Eureka"? Hardly. The announcement fell upon the scientific community with all the clamor of soft snow. The cancer establishment in particular was notified of the discovery. They ignored it.

Yet this was the first time that any bacterium had been shown to produce a substance virtually identical to a human hormone, one so similar that only very sophisticated tests could measure any difference. Furthermore, this compound was the same compound synthesized by cancer cells, spermatozoa, and the trophoblast of pregnancy. A direct link must exist between bacterial microbes and cancer cells!* The synthesis of this CG-like

*The most probable connection is transfer of DNA. A model is suggested by recent research into crown gall disease, which is a plant tumor caused by a bacterium called *Agrobacterium tumefaciens*. The bacterial cause of this plant cancer has been known since early in the century.

According to this research, the bacterium causing crown gall tumors contains a plasmid (second chromosome) that is transferred to the plant cells, where it causes the cell to pro-

substance by bacterial microbes is not to be confused with genetic engineering, which scientists are now using to create new bacterial strains that will supposedly consume oil spills and even certain metals. The discovery by Dr. Virginia Livingston-Wheeler shows that the CG synthesis by bacterial microbes isolated from cancer patients is a *naturally* occurring phenomenon. It would seem that such an outstanding discovery would have warranted a Nobel Prize, or at least a nomination, but as of this writing no such honor has resulted for Dr. Wheeler.

Besides the confirmation of Dr. Wheeler's discovery by Drs. Cohen and Strampp, two other alert scientists did not ignore Dr. Wheeler's announcement. These two men are Dr. Hernan F. Acevedo and Dr. Malcolm Slifkin. Both of them are well-known and recognized scientists, members of several of the most prestigious national and international scientific societies. Dr. Acevedo is the senior research scientist in the Division of Experimental Pathology of the Department of Laboratory Medicine, William H. Singer Memorial Research Institute of the Allegheny General Hospital, in Pittsburgh, Pennsylvania, which he joined in 1966. Since 1968, he has also held the position of adjunct assistant professor of microbiology and cell biology, Pennsylvania State Univer-

---

duce certain unusual amino acids, which are used by the bacterium. Somehow it also causes the cells to produce a tumor. Since the crown gall tumor cell has DNA from the bacteria, it is not necessary for the bacteria to remain in the tumor for the tumor to continue growth.

Just what DNA transference between bacteria and animal cells (possibly mutual) takes place is, of course, unknown.

sity. He has been principal author or coauthor of more than 100 scientific papers, abstracts, and chapters of books on such diverse topics as hormones in cancer and mesenchymal diseases, pituitary and adrenal dysfunction, biochemistry of reproduction, and hormone metabolism in normal and abnormal tissues.

Since 1964, Dr. Malcolm Slifkin has been the head of the Section of Microbiology and Immunology, Department of Laboratory Medicine, Allegheny General Hospital, and adjunct professor of microbiology, Pennsylvania State University since 1965. Since 1975, he has also been clinical assistant professor of pathology, University of Pittsburgh School of Medicine. In addition, Dr. Slifkin has authored many scientific papers in the fields of bacteriology, virology, immunology, and cancer research.

Acevedo and Slifkin were the first scientists to discover and identify chorionic gonadotropin in human spermatozoa in 1977.[1] These two scientists are also responsible for discovering that cancer cells in tissue culture of both human and animal models synthesize the CG-like material. This historical discovery was reported by Acevedo and Slifkin at the Third International Symposium on Detection and Prevention of Cancer in New York City in 1976.[2 41]

One of their most significant articles, titled "Immunohistochemical Localization of a Choriogonadotropin-like Protein in Bacteria Isolated from Cancer Patients,"[3] appeared in the April 1978 issue of *Cancer*, the official research journal of the American Cancer Society. This paper contains three important and interesting findings: (a) that fifteen strains of bacteria isolated from tissues of cancer patients show the property of synthesizing a CG-like substance; (b) that the CG-like substance was absent in noncancerous human cells and in bacteria not isolated from cancer tissues; and (c) that the CG-like protein was found on the surface of bacteria and cancerous cells.

In a later scientific paper, published in the June 1979 issue of *Infection and Immunity*, one of the official journals of the American Society of Microbiology, Acevedo, Slifkin, and associates also described the presence of the CG-like substance in a strain of bacterium called *Eubacterium lentum*.[4] This was the first time that an anaerobic bacterium (one that lives without air) had been shown to synthesize the hormonelike substance. Of further interest is the fact that this bacterium was originally isolated in France in 1938 from a rectal tumor! The bacterial strain was obtained from American Type Culture Collection, which keeps microbial strains in culture and on file for scientists to utilize in research. This discovery shows that the property of synthesizing the CG-like hormone is transmitted genetically by the bacterium from generation to generation. This publication further supported the original observation of these scientists that all bacteria exhibiting the CG-manufacturing phenomenon were isolated from cancer patients, although *not all* bacteria isolated from cancer patients exhibit this ability.

In other writings, these researchers have described that in a manner almost identical to that of cancer cells, the CG-like material is localized in the outer membrane wall of bacteria.[41 42] Furthermore, a paper by Drs. Takeshi Maruo, H. Cohen, and S. S. Koide[31] of Rockefeller University in New York City confirms that the properties of human CG and of the CG-like hormone synthesized by bacteria are similar, except for a difference in biological potency. Both exhibit the same biological activity when injected into an animal. How intriguing it would be if cultures of the microbes Dr. Scott isolated in the 1920s and that Dr. George Clark later isolated within the NIH were available today for CG testing. These are the microbes that the cancer powers have repeatedly dismissed as "contaminants."

At present, Acevedo and Slifkin are applying for grants to support their research: (a) to systematically screen bacteria of known origin for the presence of the CG-like hormone; (b) to determine the clinical frequency of the CG-like protein in bacteria isolated from patients with different types and stages of cancer as well as from noncancerous patients; (c) to determine further if any structural differences exist between bacteria that synthesize the CG-like protein and those that do not, and (d) to determine the intracellular location of the CG-like protein.

Another outstanding scientist, Dr. Gerald J. Domingue, professor of urology, microbiology, and immunology at Tulane University School of Medicine in New Orleans, has been studying for several years the role of cell-wall-defective bacteria (variants) in kidney diseases.[15 18 23 28 29] He has shown that human red blood cells are parasitized (infected) with minimal reproductive units of bacteria. This can be readily demonstrated in the blood of patients with nephritis (a disease of the kidneys) and in urine containing red blood cells from hematuric (blood in the urine) patients.[16 17 19 20 21 22]

Dr. Domingue points out that convincing circumstantial evidence indicates the possible etiologic (causative) role for these unusual microbes and/or their products in disease. Of particular significance is his finding that some of the bacterial isolates obtained from patients with nephritis and with fevers of unknown origin produce a protein similar to human chorionic gonadotropin. Therefore, it is possible that CG-producing bacteria can be isolated from noncancer patients, and such findings suggest that CG-producing bacteria may also play a role in diseases other than cancer. On the other hand, these patients may have malignancies that are not clinically detectable.

Since it has been shown that every cancer cell so far tested has CG in its membrane, it is important to determine whether there is any link between CG-producing bacteria isolated from cancer patients and CG present in cancer cells. Dr. Domingue is now injecting experimental animals with CG-producing bacteria isolated from cancer patients and from patients with kidney diseases to determine whether tumors and kidney diseases develop in these animals. He is also injecting other animals with non-CG-producing microbes as controls.

In addition, he is performing protective studies with antiserum to CG to determine if such antibodies prevent the development and spread of malignancies. Malignant cells are being exposed to antiserum derived from CG-producing bacterial vaccines and to human CG vaccines prior to injection into animals, to determine if there is a protective effect. Animals are also being immunized with human CG and with vaccines containing CG-producing bacteria prior to injection of malignant cells, to determine whether such immunized animals will be protected from development of a malignancy in comparison to nonimmunized animals.

All of this experimental work to develop the bacterial CG–cancer cell relationship and a universal vaccine against cancer is being sponsored strictly through private funding! Not one dime of money for Dr. Domingue or Dr. Acevedo and their associates is coming from the powerfully financed cancer establishment!

If it turns out that only bacterial strains that are growing in or have grown in the presence of cancer cells synthesize the CG-like protein, there can be several possible results:

1. It is necessary to reconsider the possibility that a CG-producing bacterium is the *cause* of cancer. As Acevedo writes: "An old area of research will have to be reopened and started with a fresh approach."
2. The presence of the CG hormone might be an excellent diagnostic tool to detect cancer in early stages.
3. If CG or the CG-like protein is found *only* in cancer cells, spermatozoa, trophoblasts of pregnancy, and cancer-related bacteria, this would

offer a real possibility for developing a preventive cancer vaccine!

To sum up, these basic discoveries that cancer-related bacteria and cancer cells share this remarkable ability to synthesize CG or a CG-like protein suggests to us some new and exciting facts about cancer.

First of all, if it is true that *every* cancer, whether in the bloodstream, the lymphatic system, or in organs, produces CG or a CG-like material, then from this standpoint all cancer is *one* disease, not many, as traditional teaching suggests. Of course, it may attack different parts of the body.

Second, the presence of this CG protein in every cancer cell suggests that all cancer cells have *one* mechanism, regardless of the different triggering causes such as carcinogens or radiation. Approximately 16,000 carcinogens have been identified. But now that the relationship between the bacterial microbes and the cancer cell is becoming clear, it becomes obvious how ridiculous it has been to attribute the cancer problem to all of these predisposing or weakening causes.

Third, the presence of the CG protein on the surface of every cancer cell and also on bacteria found in the cancerous tissue (including urine) of cancer patients suggests that something connects the two phenomena, although just what the relationship may be is not entirely clear. Dr. Livingston-Wheeler hypothesizes that the bacterium (she still insists that it is all one bacterium and that in its "filterable phase" it may contaminate other bacteria in the cancerous patient) invades the cell and perhaps lies dormant within it. Then some internal or external disturbance—chemical or radiation—produces a crisis in the cell, and the genetic coding of the invader either begins the synthesis of CG or somehow activates the latent gene for CG in the cell itself. Another hypothesis suggests that the bacteria somehow acquire the property of synthesizing the CG protein from the cell as it becomes a cancer cell.

Fourth, if cancer is one disease, then perhaps it can be stopped by chemically neutralizing the CG protein, with its heavy negative charge—particularly as this seems to be the mechanism by which cancer wards off the immune system.

This immensely promising line of research, with future possibilities to be discussed more fully in the next chapter, is the direct result of over eighty years of research into cancer-related bacteria—research that has been swept under the rug, denied, and mocked, while thousands of victims have died unnecessarily in the terrible pain of cancer. And it is staggering to think of what may lie ahead when this nation finally realizes what has happened since 1924.

6

Why We Can Have a Universal Cancer Vaccine

As we have said, cancer experts have long held to the belief that there are many forms of cancer. Some believe that these forms may number as many as 300. They also believe that each of these forms of cancer is a completely different disease rather than one disease. The malignant cells of one form, they say, have nothing in common with cells of another form. For example, leukemia is cancer of the blood-forming tissues, but leukemia itself is subdivided into several different types of diseases. Carcinomas are cancers of the epithelial cells, such as the skin, breast, or the cells that line the stomach. Sarcomas are cancers of connective tissue cells, for example, muscle, fat tissue, or lymph glands.

"Scientific authorities," therefore, have consistently reported to the news media and the public that there can be no "magic bullet" to cure or prevent cancer, because we are dealing with many diseases under the heading "cancer." According to this line of thinking, cancer is not a specific disease like tuberculosis or leprosy.

With the discovery that CG is found on the surface of all cancer cells thus far tested, both animal and human, this long-expounded theory of the cancer establishment—that cancer has various forms or that it is many diseases—goes out the window. In reality, the discovery and demonstration of the CG hormone provides for the first time in history a common biochemical denominator for all cancer cells.

Cancer can now be looked upon not as many diseases, but *one* disease with 300 clinical manifestations which exhibit themselves as "forms." We can explain further by an example. Tuberculosis is caused by one bacterial microbe, *Mycobacterium tuberculosis*. However, the disease can be located on the skin, lung, or other organs of the body, like cancer. Tuberculosis of the adrenal glands, for example, is called Addison's Disease. These are clinical manifestations or different forms of the same bacterial disease—tuberculosis.

CG is technically what we call an *antigen*. An antigen, by definition, is any substance that stimulates the production of antibodies or reacts with them. Antibodies are biological protein substances that "lock on" to that particular antigen associated with bacteria responsible for the disease and stop them from producing their harmful disease effects. They also attack any other foreign protein (a reason for rejection of skin grafts or organ transplants). The antigen-antibody reaction is the basis for all vaccines from polio and measles to tetanus. The Salk polio vaccine, a typical example, is made by what is known as attenuation of the polio virus, which simply means that the polio virus cultures are killed by chemical solutions like carbolic acid or formalin. The killed virus still maintains the ability to stimulate antibodies when administered in a vaccine that then protects us against the disease. The Sabin polio vaccine is prepared in a different manner by using for the vaccine live virus which has been weakened by other methods of preparation.

Because CG seems to be a universal antigen synthesized by cancer cells and bacteria from cancer patients, the possibility of a universal preventive vaccine for cancer automatically exists.

The whole purpose of any vaccine is to stimulate specific antibody formation by the immune mechanism of the individual against a particular agent—an antigen. The same antibody development sometimes results when the person acquires the disease, but this is the hard, painful way of generating specific antibodies. Vaccination is a shortcut to the antibody development process. The immune system produces specific antibodies against a disease without the body actually contracting the disease. Antibodies of one disease obviously do not protect against another disease because these are highly specific reactions.

In cancer an additional promising fact about the CG hormone being synthesized by the cancer cell is its localization in the outer wall membranes of the cell (see Figures 1-3 in Chapter 5), since this increases its vulnerability; it is somewhat like a handle to get hold of.

Myron Blume, M.D., Ph.D., Director of the Immunology Center at Mount Zion Hospital in San Francisco, California, and an expert in the field of oncology (tumors) and immunology, has this comment:

> The presence of a universal marker, one that is confirmed, will allow us to take a big step in the right direction. If that turns out to be true, it will be the first time, in my vocabulary, what could be called a breakthrough has happened in cancer in the last forty years. If you can prove that every single human cancer cell synthesizes CG, I think that would be very significant.

This statement is in reference to the already existent cancer cell, which the white blood cells cannot attack, not because they are not alerted to do so, but because they cannot approach to attack. The cancer cell must be disarmed by removing the CG hormone shield from the outer border of the cell, because the CG functions somewhat like an electric fence warding off the killer white blood cells.

We should make it clear at this point that if the outer membrane of the cancer cell can be destroyed, the cell cannot survive. It will simply break up. This principle applies to any type of cell, normal or cancerous.

Further, if the CG synthesis is a normal function in the development of the cancer cells, and solid scientific evidence indicates that it is, then obviously its formation can be prevented from happening in the first place. As we have pointed out, once the CG synthesis begins to take place in a cell, and becomes concentrated on the cell membrane, the deadly malignant process is underway. The cells have returned to a primordial or underdeveloped stage and begin to divide, completely unchallenged by the body's immune system if they accumulate or utilize the hormone in their membranes. The killer capacity of the immune mechanism of white blood cell response has been neutralized by this hormone. Moreover, the production of this hormone by both the cancer cells and the bacterial microbes disrupts the whole hormone balance system of the individual because it is no longer under control of the host glandular-hormone governing process. It throws a monkey-wrench into the delicate hormone functions because the cancer cell and bacterial microbes have set up business on their own and progress rampantly. As this process develops, the patient slowly dies because both the bacteria and cancer cells spread.

How would the proposed cancer vaccine work? Thus far Dr. Virginia Livingston-Wheeler and Dr. Hernan F. Acevedo, working independently in different parts of the nation, have shown that bacteria isolated from cancer patients are also synthesizing CG. Because the microbes share what is known in immunology as common antigenic determinants with the cancer cells, namely the CG-like substance, selected strains of these bacterial microbes can be used as the basis for the preventive vaccine. It is hoped that specific antibody formation will therefore prevent a normal cell from undergoing malignant transformation. Specific antisera against these CG-producing microbes may also bring about dramatic results, such as those obtained by Dr. Scott in the 1920s, but money is needed to explore and develop all areas of this astounding discovery about cancer cells and bacterial microbes.

To some degree, antibodies are constantly being formed by the body against normal CG, even though it is a natural body substance, but these are antibodies with very low affinity, meaning the amount of reaction is negligible.[6] Now, because of CG-producing bacteria, the potency can be raised to produce antibodies that will really do the necessary job and with the power required for immunity protection.

Dr. Acevedo has said that we can never stop the cell from its attempt at CG production because cancer is a part of life. But with the production of specific antibodies by vaccine inoculation against these microbes, the malignant transformation process by the cells will be stopped in its tracks from becoming a clinical manifestation, that is, the formation of deadly tumors and lesions which spread and kill. We will, in essence, be attacking and preventing cancer at its very roots. We will be preventing the survival of malignant cells after the cellular transformation has started to occur, therefore eliminating the presentation of the clinical disease we call cancer.

There will be no more blind shotgun approach of chemotherapy or deadly radiation in the futile attempt to try to kill cancer cells resulting in torturous and toxic effects to the already cancer-weakened patient; no more attacking an enemy cell which is not understood, because we now know how it functions, being closely and ironically linked to life itself. Cause and effect arguments are no longer important. Because of the universal CG hormone antigen, it does not matter how the cancer was produced, or as the "NBC Nightly News" reported to the nation on December 1, 1977, the antigen can be demonstrated by cancer cells regardless of how the malignant transformation was caused. It does not matter whether it was caused by chemicals or viruses. It is always present!

Dr. Acevedo has also had much experience in the field of human reproductive biochemistry. He feels that we may have not only a universal vaccine against cancer but also a vaccine against pregnancy. CG hormone is normally present, and synthesized, as we have shown, in the embryonic trophoblast and male sperm cells. If the vaccine works in preventing a cancer cell from developing, we must entertain the possibility that the CG hormone protection of the trophoblast and of the sperm cells will be destroyed upon administration of the bacterial cancer vaccine. Antibodies against a developing cancer cell would have the effect of destroying the trophoblast or preventing fertilization by destroying the sperm cell's potential.[3] As a matter of fact, in a series of reports of studies in India, reported in the February 1976 issue of *Contraception*[1] it was shown that a vaccine that neutralized the biological activity of CG significantly lowered the fertility of female rhesus monkeys. The immunization against human CG was obtained with a conjugate or combination of the beta subunit portion of the CG molecule and tetanus toxin. A preliminary report of this work was published in the January 1976 issue of the *Proceedings of the National Academy of Sciences.*[4]

The reason for this combination is that CG, by itself, will probably not stimulate specific antibody formation since it is a natural body substance. But in combination with another substance it should produce the desired antibody effect. This is why the use of CG-producing bacterial microbes will be so important in developing a universal cancer vaccine. The CG is already combined to a foreign material—the bacterial microbes—much like a steel chain connected to two cars.

To many, a pregnancy vaccine may be a godsend in itself. But if everyone took the cancer vaccine early, then the human race could possibly become extinct. How would this problem be solved? Neither Dr. Acevedo nor Dr. Livingston-Wheeler or other investigators see this as a serious problem. Of all human cancers, 90% occur after the age of 40. For those who wish to have children, the obvious solution would be to take the vaccine after age 40, because it is past usual children-bearing age. The question arises, however, as to how many people would want to take that risk. Should they have children in the hope of not developing cancer or take the vaccine before the age of 40 and not have children? Before anyone becomes too concerned, we must look at some other possibilities for the future.

Various vaccines, such as the tetanus vaccine, proven effective in preventing diseases, do not provide a lifetime protection. The vaccine shots must be renewed. If the cancer vaccine is a type requiring periodic shots to maintain immunity against the cellular CG process, then the matter of pregnancy can be regulated. Dr. Acevedo believes that we will probably need a booster type of vaccine for cancer with periodic renewal of immunity.

A study by Florence B. Seibert and Robert L. Davis of the Veterans Administration of Bay Pines, Florida, further supports the idea that the vaccine will need boosters. In a report in the *Journal of the Reticuloendothelial Society* in April 1977[2] they discuss the use of a heat-killed vaccine made from a filterable bacterial strain isolated from a mouse breast tumor. This vaccine depressed the incidence of spontaneous breast cancer about 20% from 39 to 58 weeks. However, about the sixtieth week, the effect weakened rapidly, so that by the seventy-second week, incidence of cancer in vaccinated and control mice was about the same.

On the basis of some studies, critics of the CG proposal have felt that the substance might also be present in normal tissues. Should this be the case, then a vaccine against the CG synthesis could cause harm or destroy normal and vital tissues, for example, if CG was *normally* present in some heart muscle cells. Specific antibodies against CG would seek out and destroy those cells, causing irreparable damage or even death. However, most recent studies suggest that the substance which supposedly reacted in the experiments on normal tissue, other than male sperm cells and the trophoblast of pregnancy, was not genuine CG or a CG-like substance but rather a common body protease that can mimic CG in certain concentrations and certain diagnostic methods.[5] Therefore, when it comes right down to extremely meticulous biochemistry, the opposition has lost their final argument by the absolute demonstration of positive, scientific facts.

In light of the CG-like substance produced by the microbes and cancer cells, the possibility of cancer being a low-grade contagious disease must be considered. This too has been dismissed as nonsense by the cancer establishment in the past. The evidence of leukemia outbreaks in schools in New Jersey and the epidemic levels of cancer in China and elsewhere can no longer be passed off as coincidence. The possibility, if not probability, of cancer being an infectious, contagious disease was pointed out by some of the early investigators we have discussed in the first part of this book, but they were crushed for proposing such nonsense. Now the epidemic increase of cancer faces us with this same evidence once again which simply cannot be ignored in view of the demonstrable link between CG-producing bacteria and the cancer cell which duplicates the same process.

7

Other Possibilities

Although the production of an anti-cancer vaccine is, as we have demonstrated, a scientifically sound possibility, the actual production and testing of such a vaccine is likely to be several years away, under the best circumstances. The time could be shortened by a crash program, of course, but this is unlikely because of the politics and behind-the-scene intrigue of cancer research. This is perhaps the biggest obstacle ahead.

In the meantime, the phenomenon of CG as a surface antigen of every cancer cell leads to possibilities of very early diagnosis and therapy that might well be of primary importance. For example, further confirmation of the presence of CG in cancer cells has been published in a recent paper in *Science*[1] by David M. Goldenberg and associates, which discusses a use of CG as an early diagnostic tool.

If radioactive antibodies to human CG are injected into a human body, the antibodies will travel to the site of CG and, in layman's terms, stick there. As we have seen, the most likely site will be the surfaces of cancer cells. If such a site of CG is in the body, a total body scan with a gamma-ray scintillation camera attached to a computer will detect concentrations of radioactivity and give their precise locations in the body. By this means the experimenters are able to detect cancers that are not detectable by X-ray, ultrasonography, venography, or CT scanning. The development of purer antibodies, by techniques to be described, makes this by far the most important diagnostic tool ever discovered. This method of carrying material to a cancer site might also be used for more precise use of chemotherapy agents, as Goldenberg and associates suggest.

The success of the antiserum of Scott, Glover, White, and others in the 1920s and 1930s was probably due to antibodies against CG rather than antibodies to cancer-related bacteria, although these bacterial microbes became the vehicle or instruments for bringing about the specific reaction which combated cancer cells. While the production of quantities of high purity human CG antibody is expensive and difficult, a new technology suggests a therapy based on the use of larger quantities of antibody to the CG coating on cancer cells.

This technique is known as the production of "hybridomas," developed in 1976 by Cesar Milstein and Georges Kohler of the British Medical Council Laboratory of Molecular Biology. It involves injecting mice with antigen and then fusing antibody manufacturing cells with certain types of cancer cells. The result, called a hybridoma, can then be cloned, and the resultant generations can reproduce without limit, thus making possible large quantities of specific antibodies uncontaminated with other substances.

Already "monoclonal" antibodies (that is, made from a hybridoma) to human CG are available commercially, although they are not licensed for use in human beings. An unpublished paper by J.A. Kellen and associates[2] states that the use of an antiserum against CG on rat cancer cells resulted in a great decrease in metastasis or spread of cancer cells. More study should be given to use of larger quantities of pure antibody in combating CG at the cancer site, perhaps combined with immune system stimulation.

Chemotherapy is another idea that might be strengthened based upon the demonstrable fact of the presence of CG on cancer cell surfaces. Present chemotherapy agents are extremely toxic with devastating side effects. But now that the cancer cell is understood in relation to CG, effective, nontoxic agents may possibly be developed to work in conjunction with a specific CG vaccine and antiserum.

In other words, the universal presence of CG on the surface of cancer cells is in a real sense the "open sesame" to an effective end to cancer in our time. New diagnostic tools, more effective therapies, and above all, a preventive vaccine against cancer in humans and animals are distinct possibilities.

The immediate question is how can the cancer establishment ignore this information? And another question: why are millions of dollars being spent on projects like Interferon, which does not begin to have the scientific foundation that CG and the bacterial microbes have?

The answers to these questions will be given in the next chapters, which tell of the deep and often dogmatic conservatism of science and the way in which cancer research is funded and directed. As we proceed through these sections of the book, we will gain a greater understanding of why Dr. Donald Kennedy, the former director of the federal Food and Drug Administration has described the "war on cancer" as a "medical Vietnam."[4]

8

Modern Science and New Ideas

In the summer of 1976, the nation's bicentennial year, the American Legion held its convention in Philadelphia and entered the history of medicine. On July 27, the first Legionnaire died of what was to be called Legionnaire's Disease. Of the some 160 men who got the disease, 29 died.

The attempts to find out what went wrong in Philadelphia make a remarkable story or perhaps a grim comedy. For months the theories came in: virus, possibly from pigeons, Lassa fever, a fungus, swine flu (another fiasco of that year), bootleg liquor, nickel carbynol poisoning, and phosphene gas. Finally, as the result of a hunch by two alert scientists, Dr. Charles Shephard and microbiologist Joseph McDade of the National Disease Control Center in Atlanta, Georgia, the cause turned out to be a bacterium of the rickettsia family, the same type of bacterium that causes Rocky Mountain Spotted Fever. The bacterium likes a moist environment and was probably in the air-conditioning system. Since this bacteria is smaller than usual—actually between normal bacteria and viruses in size—and is hard to culture (cancer-related bacteria also have been hard to culture, by the way), we should not be too critical of the slowness in isolating the culprit. Yet, we must wonder if the long delay in finding the cause of Legionnaire's Disease was not partly due to the fact that in the 1970s and 1980s it is unpopular to believe that a bacterium can cause a new or unrecognized disease! Some scientists now believe that what has been labeled Legionnaire's Disease may have been with us for years, killing thousands of people annually, but had been unrecognized. As far as academic medicine is concerned, diseases today are caused by viruses or chemicals, two favorites of the cancer establishment. Bacteria went out with Pasteur and Koch.

Most of us grow up with the myth that most questions about the natural world have been answered and that laboratories of brilliant young Dr. Arrowsmiths are busy searching in the few corners of mystery left. Actually, things are not quite so simple.

In his classic book on science, *The Structure of Scientific Revolutions*,[5] Thomas Kuhn says that at any given time in any science, the major researchers share what he calls a "paradigm" or model of the science, which includes "laws, theory, applications, and instrumentation." For example, in Newton's time, the paradigm of light was material corpuscles. Most of the experimentation under this paradigm was to demonstrate that light did in fact exert pressure on solid bodies. This paradigm was succeeded by the transverse wave theory, which provided experimenters a vision that led to some valuable insights. The physics of today tells us that light is photons, which sometimes act like particles, sometimes like waves. Under a paradigm or model, the *acceptable* research is only in those areas that fit under the particular model of the science or slice of the universe studied by the science.

Eventually, new discoveries will not fit the model, and the model changes, usually with ill grace and disbelief on the part of senior conservative practitioners of the science, who have firmly entrenched views.

Although the development of paradigms is very useful in setting limits to inquiry and stimulating important research, it also tends to reinforce the natural conservatism of scientists and their tunnel vision, making the consideration of new phenomena extremely difficult regardless of the provable facts that demonstrate the new phenomena. The inventive scientist is shoved out of official circles because he is not part of the conservative thinking of the "in" clique. The whole area becomes somewhat of a mutual admiration society, placing emphasis on who the scientist is, who he knows, and the prestige of the institution where he works. It is an ideal setup for self-perpetuation with no end in sight.

When we go back to Scott and his early experiments and the story of how he was virtually silenced by colleagues and other institutions of science, we tend to classify his critics as villains akin to narrow-minded inquisitors silencing Galileo. But basically the problem is that the paradigms of cancer have not usually allowed the concept that it is an infectious disease or that bacteria could have anything to do with it, although the very pattern of cancer dictates that it is infectious, starting at one source and spreading to distant points in the body. In so far as they were educated in the models or paradigms of the day, most doctors and researchers of Scott's day (or ours) were unable to transcend the model of their science to include something that did not fit. The persistent emphasis of the National Cancer Institute and American Cancer Society on chemotherapy, carcinogens, and viruses does not occur because of wickedness or atypical myopia on the part of those who give out the money. In part, at least, the blindness to new discoveries comes from the fact that the paradigm of cancer is the picture we have described before—perhaps 300 diseases "caused" by carcinogenic chemicals and possibly viruses, best treated by surgery, chemotherapy, and radiation. Bacterial microbes that have now been identified as being CG producers isolated from cancer patients have been condemned as being contaminants, thus further reducing in everyone's mind the possibility that cancer could be an infectious disease. This closed universe of science can be shown by many other examples of repression of major discoveries.

Let us examine the work of a pioneer in cancer diagnosis, Dr. George Nicholas Papanicolaou (1883–1962), the developer of the famous Pap Test.[3] He began his research with guinea pigs, then with the reproductive system of women, as early as 1910. His work led him to feel that the cervical smear, examined with stains and the use of the microscope, was a valuable and reliable way to diagnose cancer of the uterine cervix. He published a paper in 1928, about the time that Scott and Glover were working on cancer-related bacteria. Since pathologists were convinced that only biopsy (examination of tissue removed from the organ) had value for diagnosis, his ideas were not seriously considered until 1943, 15 years later! His ideas and techniques did not fit within the accepted principles of the time. If it had not been for the fact that other researchers were now on the same trail, the work of Papanicolaou might have continued to languish. Indeed, it was not until 1948, 20 years later, that the American Cancer Society began actively to promote the test. It appeared to be a new technique to the public, although it was far from being new, only unrecognized. Many women's lives were lost in the years between 1928 and 1948 because the scientific world ignored this useful screening test. The scientific frame of mind was not yet ready for its acceptance when Dr. Papanicolaou announced his discovery in 1928.

The story of Jonas Salk is even more instructive in examining this phenomenon.[2] Almost everyone believes that Salk got his discovery and development of the polio vaccine out to the world like magic, with enthusiastic acceptance from his peers. As Salk progressed in his study of polio viruses, he became convinced that the vaccine that would produce the most antibodies most safely was a killed-virus vaccine. This was contrary to the model of polio established by his respected peers. Pressure from traditional virus scientists like Dr. Albert Sabin, who believed that only a live-virus vaccine could be effective, and Dr. John Enders, Nobel prize winner for growing polio virus in foreskins, was heavy indeed. Enders, in fact, is reported to have accused Salk of quackery,[2] the term that at times has embraced the most profound truth and the most utter nonsense. Salk was challenging the very foundation and beliefs of the polio establishment.

In spite of the fact that the Salk vaccine was very successful, successful beyond the expectations of the developer and his associates, the Sabin live-virus vaccine, prepared by the Charles Pfizer pharmaceutical manufacturing company, was promoted vigorously by the AMA for private vaccination even before it had been licensed for public use. The AMA went right on promoting live vaccine as though Salk had never existed! This was in spite of clear evidence that the Salk vaccine was effective wherever it was given. At the time of Salk's discovery of the polio vaccine he was a relatively unknown scientist. His fame skyrocketed overnight much to the dismay of his peers. He was accused of "allowing" his name to become attached to the polio vaccine as the press became aware of his discovery—a serious violation of the closed-circuit code laid down by these peers. This was professional jealousy at its worst. Jonas Salk was never awarded the Nobel Prize, which he so richly deserved for ridding the world of polio. To this day he has never been nominated to the National Academy of Sciences, which is an invitational honor bestowed by its members. Although the Salk polio vaccine is available in most countries of the world, it is not available in the United States.

We can call up many other names, such as Semmelweis (1818–1865), who practically eradicated childbirth fever in Vienna by having the students wash their hands after coming from dissection to deliver babies! His reward was to be driven from Vienna in 1849. His vindication came much later.[9]

The story of penicillin is similar.[7] The Scottish bacteriologist, Sir Alexander Fleming, discovered in 1928 that products of the cultures of *Penicillium*, a fungus mold, had an inhibitive effect on the growth of some bacteria. It was not until World War II that its beneficial merits in fighting infected wounds were recognized and utilized routinely. Had it not been for the war, perhaps many more years would have passed before it gained acceptance.

The inherent conservatism of science is further enhanced by the institution of peer review. Most scientific journals, for example, which are the only way new ideas can get a hearing, are not run like commercial magazines. Scientific journals have a stable of experts who review the articles for scientific accuracy and worth—or perhaps, more accurately, how well the proposed scientific papers fit into what the referees consider to be the acceptable ways of doing the science. Ideas different from the referee's rarely get the nod. Old students, friends, and people who do research as the referee does it get published, regardless of the failure of these ideas from past experience. Again, who you are, who you know, and the prestige of your institution get top billing. Since this system is also used in giving research grants, the investigator has to face the fact that peer groups sitting in judgment may well be honest and earnest seekers after truth, but also people with narrowness of vision and a dogmatic certainty.[4]

An example of the frustration that peer review, at least as presently conducted, can cause because of human factors and bias can be shown in the experiences of Dr. Hernan Acevedo and his associates whose work we have discussed.

Early in 1977 the Pathology B Study Section of the National Institutes of Health evaluated a proposal by Drs. Acevedo and Slifkin to investigate the presence of CG in a wide range of cancer cells and tissues. All these scientists wanted to do was to expand their studies to see if it is one hundred percent positive. In the critique section of the evaluation, several points were brought up, some of them directly contradictory. For example, the reviewers said that the "methodology appears to have been worked out, and there are sufficient preliminary data . . . to indicate that the project can be accomplished." However, in later sections, the techniques used were questioned on various grounds. The overall evaluation was approval of the grant with a cut budget and the subsequent assignment of a low priority number, a real slap in the face, which, of course, killed the grant. Why should anyone be afraid to see if the CG discovery about the bacterial microbes or cancer cells is valid? The worst that could have happened would be to find that it is not valid.

A revised proposal was evaluated in October of 1977. Here the review group complained that the project was not imaginative and not very clear.

Again, however, they advocated funding the project but with another low priority number. But this behind-the-scene intrigue goes further.

Not satisfied by this reaction, Dr. Acevedo asked that the proposal be submitted to the Allergy and Immunology Study Section for review. After all, this does come under immunology if an eventual vaccine may result. There were more months of delay before a response was forthcoming.

This group turned down the proposal on the grounds that "*the authors have virtually accomplished the goals of their proposal.*" This panel, as the Pathology B Study Section, was composed of about 14 experts in biochemistry and immunology from various universities and research centers around the nation, who are consultants to the Division of Research Grants of the National Institutes of Health. In their opinion the CG synthesis by *all* cancer cells had been adequately demonstrated! Stated another way, the biochemical common denominator of *all* cancer cells had been found with no further work necessary to scientifically demonstrate this historical discovery. Still, there was no announcement made to the press or Congress to make them aware of this major breakthrough on the cancer cell. Why? A universal common denominator has been acknowledged by recognized experts and the discovery has been greeted with little or no enthusiasm, or should we say contempt? This panel, too, felt the project lacked creativity, but this was not the purpose of Acevedo's and Slifkin's scientific paper. It was clear from their proposal that this was considered basic science necessary for further work, not innovation.

Since the Pathology B and the Allergy and Immunology Study Sections disagreed, Dr. Arthur Upton, who was then Director of the NCI, asked the Division of Research Grants to provide a third review section, which was "not provided with summary statements from previous reviews . . . in order to avoid the introduction of bias." Let the reader clearly see this picture. A school child could see the folly of the setup that was to follow. Here we have two different opinions from two different review sections composed of regarded scientific "experts." A very embarrassing situation to say the least. It is little wonder that no announcement was made to the press or to Congress about the discovery of the universal CG synthesis by all cancer cells. Had these two review panels been hauled up before a Congressional subcommittee for indepth investigation and questioning we might have the cancer vaccine project well underway by now. But the acknowledged CG discovery slipped right by members of Congress who have been led to believe anything the NCI hands them and who are busy men and women who simply do not have the time to keep tabs on what is happening in NIH study sections.

As expected, the third review turned out to be nothing more than a kangaroo court for Dr. Acevedo and his associates. He was in a Catch 22 position, and the entire embarrassing situation was white-washed. On this review panel, for instance, was a scientist whose basic idea about CG, as Acevedo wrote to Dr. Upton following the meeting, would be proved wrong if his CG hypothesis were proved correct. Likewise, on the special team was a scientist from the Laboratory of Immunodiagnosis of the NCI. One of his papers had been reviewed unfavorably in Dr. Acevedo's proposal.

Had, at that time, a Congressional subcommittee brought Dr. Acevedo before them, they would have seen the most beautiful color slides imaginable, photographs taken under the microscope, that clearly show the localization of the CG hormone in every type of cancer cell and various strains of bacterial microbes isolated from cancer patients. Explained on a layman's level of understanding, any congressperson could have seen the significance of what will undoubtedly be regarded by historians as one of the greatest medical discoveries of all time. The CG hormone synthesis permits a scientific first whereby the cancer cell can be defined as to its nature and its specific biochemistry as demonstrated by highly sophisticated biochemical techniques.

A proposal by Dr. Acevedo and his associates to investigate bacterial strains for the production of CG suffered the same fate in the NIH, since it was reviewed for the first time by the same Special Study Section, which again showed little understanding and certainly no sympathy for this proposal, in spite of its intrinsic importance to the study of cancer.

The absolute power of the National Institutes of Health complex over research has been enhanced by Congressional inquiries into claimed cancer "cures" like Laetrile, since the "cures" have usually proved to be unsuccessful. This has created an atmosphere in which ideas like those discussed in this book are likely to be dismissed abruptly. Obviously, the public picture of cancer research, especially with so many millions of dollars being spent on it, is entirely different from what goes on behind-the-scenes.

What is needed in the world of science is some realization of what Alfred North Whitehead called the "fallacy of dogmatic finality," the belief that we know the limits of the universe and believe that our knowledge is eternal and everlasting, that we know all that is important about cancer or black holes or light or time or viruses, that anyone who thinks unconventional thoughts is a crackpot or a charlatan.

Whitehead said:

> The universe is vast. Nothing is more curious than the self-satisfied dogmatism with which mankind at each period of its history cherishes the delusion of the finality of existing modes of knowledge.[8]

Jacob Bronowski, the fine humanistic tracer of human progress, in talking about Germany in the 1930s and the Heisenberg Principle of Uncertainty in physics, extends the concept into another area:

> Science has progressed step by step, the most successful enterprise in the ascent of man, because it has understood that the exchange of information between man and nature, and man and man, can only take place with a certain tolerance. But second, I also use the word passionately about the real world. All knowledge, all information between human beings,

> can only be exchanged within a play of tolerance. And that is true whether the exchange is in science or in literature, or in religion, or in politics, or even in any form of thought that aspires to dogma. It is a major tragedy of my lifetime and yours that, here in Göttingen, scientists were refining to the most exquisite precisions the Principle of Tolerance, and turning their back on the fact that all around them tolerance was crashing to the ground beyond repair.[1]

For a final testimony, let us turn to the witness of that most humanistic of physicians, Sir William Osler. In a speech before the Royal College of Physicians on October 18, 1906, entitled "The Growth of Truth Illustrated in the Discovery of the Circulation of the Blood," Osler paraphrases William Harvey in exhorting "the Fellows and Members to study out the secrets of Nature by way of experiment; and lately, for the honor of the profession, to continue in love and affection among ourselves."[6]

Science is truly a great adventure of the human mind. Our society with its toys and its impressive inventions is a living example of the power of science to transform the world. How unfortunate that the adventure is often marred by prejudice, self-satisfaction, pettiness, and intolerance of a kind that scientists would consider beneath contempt in religion or philosophy or politics but which seems to be most reasonable common sense in their own branch of science.

Throughout this book, we have been chronicling the research of intelligent, often gifted men and women who have tried time and again to get a hearing in the world of institutionalized science.

Their case is far from unique, and possibly many other areas of research which might be beneficial to humanity are hidden because they too have never had a hearing. The First Amendment to the Constitution guarantees us freedom of speech, but not necessarily a platform on which to speak. It is probably our loss that there are not more platforms where daring and unconventional research could have a voice.

9

Money and Cancer: Does Anyone Really Want to Conquer This Disease?

We have seen that the institutionalization of science, however productive it has been, tends to make it inflexible, conservative, and often virtually deaf to new or unconventional ideas. This situation is further complicated by the conditions under which cancer research is presently financed and sponsored.

Two organizations dominate cancer research today: the American Cancer Society (ACS), the largest of the privately funded health organizations, and the National Cancer Institute (NCI).

The ACS was founded in 1913 by laymen and physicians to educate the public and encourage it to seek medical advice. By the 1940s it had developed into an interesting coalition of medical professionals and leading laymen from industry, business, and the Republican Party. Since 1945, the group has used professional fund-raising techniques that have kept the ACS the most affluent disease organization in the United States. Part of this fund-raising technique is fear, causing many people to believe cancer is the number-one disease, despite the fact that it is still behind cardio-vascular diseases as a killer. The annual ACS fund-raising drive is usually headed by a well-known celebrity as honorary chairman to bring attention to the drive.[15]

The NCI was founded in 1937, the first of the National Institutes of Health, a U.S. government agency. By no coincidence, the two organizations have been much influenced in their thinking about cancer by the ideas of the practitioners—the gynecologists, the radiologists, the surgeons, and the pathologists—many of whom have sat on the boards of the ACS and NCI, sometimes on both boards at the same time.

In contrast, outside of these groups researchers in basic science have had little or no influence in changing the directions of the ACS-NCI and have been ignored or actively discouraged. We have only to examine the recent occurrences described to see this policy. This was certainly noticeable in the fight for more money for NCI, as we shall see.

In 1971, largely because of the advanced planning and strong efforts by ACS officers like Mary Lasker, a long-time cancer worker and member of the prestigious Lasker Foundation, Congress began to put some real money into the cancer enterprise. Between 1937 and 1971, the total government expenditures on cancer research totaled only 2 billion dollars, while the year's appropriation in 1971 was estimated at about 200 million dollars, one-tenth of the total expenditure during the previous thirty-four years.

A panel of consultants proposed three things:

1. that a new autonomous government agency—the National Cancer Authority—be established to conquer cancer immediately.
2. that a comprehensive national plan for the conquest of cancer be developed, utilizing "structured research" in place of "creative research."
3. that the budget for cancer research be immediately doubled to 400 million dollars with yearly increases until it reached 800 million dollars by 1976.[15]

As a model, the group was looking at NASA, which, starting late in the face of a Russian headstart, managed to get men on the moon, albeit at great expense. By analogy, they believed that a similar semiautonomous agency with plenty of money could conquer cancer.

One important difference between the space program and the cancer program, however, was the state of knowledge. In the case of the space program, the scientific basis was well known, the problems being to apply existing science and invent new hardware. The state of knowledge in cancer research was far from that in astrophysics and propulsion systems. As a matter of fact, more than one medical scientist has said that the major obstacle to our defeating major disease is our *ignorance of the basic biological facts of health and disease.*[8] As Dr. Ernest W. Siward of the University of Rochester School of Medicine and Dentistry was quoted in *The Christian Science Monitor*:

> The impression often obtained from medical scientists and from the press is that the scientific knowledge on

> which medical practice is based is vast. If we look carefully, however, it appears more as an archipelago of knowledge in a sea of ignorance. And the efficaciousness in medical practice of what we think we know has never in fact been substantiated.[18]

Considering the small effect this great flood of money has had on the conquest of cancer, we cannot but be amazed at the innocence of those who supposed that money alone would do the task, particularly considering the "structured" research directions of the ACS-NCI.

Both groups have consistently preferred to sponsor clinical research instead of basic biological research on the rationale that we cannot wait until the fundamental knowledge is in before we begin to treat cancer patients. One result has been that the NCI became the first Public Health Institute to use contracts with organizations instead of peer-screened grants to individuals. This practice allowed them to push certain research lines hard—carcinogens, chemotherapy, and virus research—while other research, as we have seen, often goes begging in spite of proof positive evidence that can be demonstrated as to the function of the cancer cell.

Big money and this kind of directed research have had a great deal to do with what kind of research is really done. If you were a young Ph.D. in biological science and wanted to get hardware and housekeeping money for your college or your research institute and wanted to get publications in scientific journals to further your career, you would certainly want to do research where the money is, say in carcinogens, viruses, or chemotherapy, because these are the accepted avenues to follow. You would be a fool or an incurable idealist if you went into cell metabolism or bacteria or some other unpopular basic field where money is not readily available.

There is no question that the vast amount of government money (not by defense standards, perhaps, but by medical research standards) has actually *narrowed* the scope of cancer research with the result of a vast expenditure of effort, the consequences of which for human knowledge or for cancer have been slight indeed. A quick survey of the cancer papers in many medical journals will convince any reader who can plow through them that much research is trivial or of no consequence, except that some of the experiments, such as repetition of carcinogen testing on hamster testicles, are bizarre enough to belong in the third book of *Gulliver's Travels*, the voyage to the ridiculous scientific anti-Utopia of La Puta.

The more money spent and the more that is demanded naturally brings the conclusion that cancer is an extremely complicated disease with no genuine clues as to what the disease is or how its biochemistry functions.

A long battle in Congress preceded the big funding. The question of the autonomy of the proposed new cancer agency was a major source of disagreement, with most of the scientific community opposed to the ACS proposal for an independent agency.

The final compromises resulted in a National Advisory Cancer Council with twenty-three members, five ex-officio (National Institutes of Health), no more than twelve physicians and no more than eight laymen. The appointees to the NACC and the head of the reorganized NCI are presidential appointees.

As Richard Rettig has pointed out, from the beginning, the National Cancer Program has been the target of intense criticism.[15] Scientists have stated correctly that not enough scientific information exists to support a large research program and that increased funds for cancer dries up money for other research in biology. Pragmatic congressmen have opposed pure research at the expense of immediate results. Environmentalists have complained that too much attention is addressed to cures, too little toward preventive control of the environment.[8]

Internal problems have plagued the agency since its inception also partly because of the sheer magnitude of the operation. For example, a report of the Comptroller General of the United States dated February 10, 1978[6] tells what is probably a fairly typical case of misuse of federal funds by the Eppley Institute. The Eppley Institute is part of the University of Nebraska and a component of the Nebraska University Medical Center. Its director is Dr. Phillipe Shubik, a member of the National Cancer Advisory Board, who has constantly been opposed to such environmental issues as banning insecticides like chlorodane and heptachlor and the Memoranda of Alert, by which NCI warned the community of early findings in its bioassay program, which tested chemicals to which people are likely to be exposed. He also has appeared at NCI meetings as a representative of industry, including Procter and Gamble, Royal Crown Cola, Abbott Laboratories, General Foods, Colgate Palmolive, the Flavor and Extract Manufacturers Association, and the Calorie Control Council.[8]

Employing biologists, chemists, pathologists, biochemists, and epidemiologists, the Institute took over in 1968 (when the head researcher and his staff came to Omaha) research originally begun in 1950 at the University of Chicago. The work at the Institute has been in testing suspected carcinogen chemicals, developing methods of detecting carcinogens, studying the mechanisms of carcinogenesis, applying the studies to human beings, and training younger investigators.

In 1968, the year the group moved to Nebraska, a direct contract with the NCI was made for 6.4 million dollars. This was renewed in 1973 for a period to end in 1978, the cost being 16.4 million. A further 3-year extension in 1977 added 3.6 million dollars, making a grand total of 26 million dollars!

During this period, the Eppley Institute undertook about 154 projects involving environmental carcinogens, foods, additives, selected pharmaceuticals, coal tar, and petroleum combustion products. Important discoveries listed by the comptroller's report include three: (a) discovery that ascorbate (Vitamin C) will inhibit nitrates—used to keep meat preserved and rosy red—from forming carcinogens in the body; (b) discovery that niridazole, a drug used to treat tropical schistosomal disease, is a potent carcinogen; and (c) the development of models for testing potential carcinogens on a variety of cancers. The rest of the research apparently has resulted in little else of discernible value in prevention or treatment of cancer.

Moreover, in examining the practices of the Eppley Institute, the Comptroller General's investigators found the following:

1. The NCI did not "properly or diligently" administer a contract with the Eppley Institute.
2. Technical review of work done was conducted by an ad hoc rather than a standing committee, and recommendations of the committee were not heeded.
3. The argument for a noncompetitive contract award on the grounds of its uniqueness was "weak and not totally supported by fact."

In addition, the investigators found that travel money used by the Eppley staff was not properly controlled, that supplies purchased with NCI contract funds were used on non-contract projects and that leave by professional staff was not handled adequately.[5] The report also comments on the practice of continuing projects not part of current contracts, and on the inadequacy of reporting.

When one considers the total NCI budget every year, (1 billion dollars, 1980–1981), the possibility of other mismanagement and corruption on this scale is highly probable.

Cancer research has been particularly prone to conflicts of interest and problems of industrial ties. In 1960, long before the elevated funding, another United States Comptroller General's Report[7] dealt with price-fixing problems with 5-FU, one of the first and still commonly used cancer chemotherapy agents.

5-FU, otherwise known as 5-Fluorouracil, was discovered by Dr. Charles Heidelberger of the University of Wisconsin along with an employee of Hoffman-La Roche pharmaceutical. They obtained a patent in 1957. Heidelberger assigned his patent rights to the American Cancer Society because some ACS funds went into the development of the chemical.

As part of its program to supply chemicals to grantees for laboratory studies and clinical evaluations, the National Institutes of Health awarded four price-fixing contracts for production and delivery of 5-FUDR (a chemical cousin of 5-FU) amounting to $60,000 for one kilogram in June 1958, an additional $60,000 for a kilogram in September, $450,000 for 5 kilograms in October, and $145,000 for 5 kilograms in June 1959.

What this meant in effect was that while the drug manufacturing company gained in experience and efficiency, their costs went down rather dramatically, so that by 1959 the profit on the drug had risen from a reasonable 10.6 percent to some 32.6 percent. Considering that the NCI was performing the basic research on the drug for the company, it was also subsidizing the company fairly heavily, using the taxpayers' dollars.

In a report to Representative David R. Obey, entitled *The Objectives of the Cancer Control Program and the National Cancer Institutes Administration of Program Contracts*, released July 13, 1980, the General Accounting Office examined five contracts of the Cancer Control Program of the National Cancer Institute. The Cancer Control Program was designed to apply research through demonstration projects and to sponsor programs of prevention, diagnosis, and counseling. The 5 contracts totalled 10.3 million dollars out of about 216 million allocated for contracts in the past five fiscal years.

The examined contracts were awarded to the Universities of Arizona and Louisiana, Illinois Cancer Council, New York State Department of Health, Health Research, Inc., and Texas Chest Foundation-East Texas Chest Hospital. Contracts with Louisville and Texas were for model programs for preventing cancer caused by exposure to vinyl-polyvinyl-chloride and to asbestos. The Arizona contract dealt with controlling breast cancer, the New York study with cervical cancer, and the Illinois contract with controlling breast cancer.

The report states that in four out of five of these contracts randomly chosen for close examination, the NCI did not correctly manage the contracts. More specifically, the GAO states the following about the contracts:

1. Recommendations of review committees were not followed up or enforced.
2. Review committees received no feedback on the implementation of their recommendations.
3. Demonstration projects, supposedly continued by communities when federal funding ended, were not followed up as to their continuation.
4. Increases in funding (up to triple funding)

were made without mandated changes in the program plan.

5. Contractors did not accomplish many of the tasks set forth in the contracts.

In three of the contracts, the following accomplishment ratios were shown:

Contractor	*Tasks to Be Accomplished*	*Accomplished*	*Cost*
Louisville	11	4	2.4 million
New York	9	2	1.5 million
Tyler, Texas	13	2	2.1 million

Incidentally, 20 research institutions receive 50% of all the NCI funding for cancer research annually!

While the GAO suggests that some present techniques and situations are improved, it also suggests that the random sample is indicative of the total of the NCI contracts, a fact disputed, of course, by the NCI. However, this kind of carelessness, if not outright corruption, is, as we have seen, typical of former investigations discussed here.

Connections between industry and the NCI have undoubtedly had their effect on certain policies. Benno Schmidt, who has been chairman of the Cancer Panel of the NCI for several years, has ties to the oil, steel, and chemical industries. On the Advisory Board are people like Elmer Bobst of Warner Lambert pharmaceutical manufacturing company, Clark Wescoe of the pharmaceutical manufacturing industry, and Dr. Jonathan Rhodes, chairman of Pennwalt Corporation, a manufacturer of chemicals. This heavy influence of industry and pharmaceutical manufacturing companies further encourages the type of research that profits industry and deemphasizes information that causes problems for industry.[8] The latest promotion for Interferon as a possible effective agent against cancer was greatly influenced by how much profit would be gained from its manufacture.

Many employees of the NCI are unhappy with the agency because of the lack of scientific acumen on the part of some of its administrators and the little progress made so far. Dr. Dean Burk, with whom one of the authors has been in periodic contact, was director of the Biochemistry Section of the NCI for years and an outspoken critic of NCI policies right to the time of his retirement a few years ago. Dr. Burk wrote several open letters to the directors of the NCI but received little cooperation for his efforts.

One of the interesting features of the cancer effort is the part played by the American Cancer Society, which is the spokesman or main propagandist for the cancer establishment. The exchange of personnel between the ACS and the NCI (as in the case of Dr. Frank Rauscher, who in 1977, went from a $40,000 per year job with NCI to a $75,000 per year job with ACS) and the placement of some persons on boards of both certainly make them closely tied organizations, regardless of the legal separation.[5]

Certainly the most notorious example of their joint action was the 1973–1978 Breast Cancer Detection Demonstration Project, touted rightly at the time as "the greatest public relations thing the NCI and the ACS have ever done."[9] NCI furnished about 85 percent of the 54.6 million dollar project! The object was to "mobilize" some 100,000 women per year for thermography, X-ray mammography, and physical examinations. Scientific objections, particularly to the X-ray part of the testing, were ignored and certainly not reported in the press. To quote Ruth Rosenbaum, from her excellent research published in the now defunct *New Times Magazine*:

> Meanwhile, not even the simplest precautions were taken to keep x-ray exposure to a minimum. A report by Ralph Nader's Research Group showed that 33—or 55—percent of the x-ray machines surveyed in 1975 emitted more than the acceptable limit of 2.5 Roentgens per film.[10]

Although statistics indicated that the testing would not be very useful for women under 50, the age dropped to 35, and the American College of Radiologists wanted it dropped still further to the age of 30!

The fact is, and this was no surprise to many biomedical scientists, the screening program probably will cause many more cancers than it detects. (By causing, we mean in relation to the documentation of this book, a weakening or predisposition that triggers the bacterial-cancer cell relationship.) As NCI assistant director Bayard Morrison is reported to have said, "We didn't do our homework," one of the classic examples of understatement of all time.

While all of this was going on, objections were not publicized, and no indication was given to women that *any* risk was involved, until May 1977. In August of 1977 the NCI finally sent a letter suggesting that the screening be restricted to women *over* 50. The response in the medical community was to ignore the letter as an example of more governmental interference in free enterprise. Originally, women *under* 50 made up 50 percent of the participants in the ACS-NCI Screening Project. Six months after strict guidelines were issued, 75 percent of women *under* 50 were still being X-rayed!

As one might expect, this was not publicly recognized for the mismanagement of funds and total irresponsibility toward medical patients it was. The press, of course, went right along with anything the cancer establishment said was the way to go for cancer. As a matter of fact, the 1977 yearly report of the ACS[1] has a glowing tribute to this wonderful program with a picture of a *young* black woman getting a breast X-ray!

The ACS itself has engaged in some rather peculiar practices. For example, one of the standing committees of the ACS is the Committee on Unproven Cancer Management, which works hand-in-glove with the AMA Committee on Quackery, both of which in the words of Ruth Rosenbaum "form a network of vigilantes prepared to pounce on anyone who promotes a cancer therapy that runs against their substantial prejudices and profits."[16] Certainly the genuine quacks must be kept under control, which no one disputes, but from the time of Dr. Michael J. Scott, some promising ideas (along with some obvious foolish ones) have been buried alive. From time to time, as in the case of Dr. Bradford Coley's work with infection as a stimulus to the immune system, the establishment has had to resurrect some of the victims of intolerance.

Another activity of the American Cancer Society has been the chipping away of the Delaney Amendment to the Food, Drug, and Cosmetic Act of 1958. The Amendment states,

> "No additive shall be claimed to be safe if it is found to induce cancer when ingested by man or animal, or if it is found after tests which are appropriate for the evaluation of safety of food additives to induce cancer in man or animals."[8]

In the great saccharin controversy of 1977 the Delaney Amendment was invoked on the basis of about three decades of research with animals and human beings which showed a statistical correlation between saccharin and bladder cancer.

The actions of some officials have been inconsistent, to say the least. For example, in June 1977, when Dr. Rauscher was contacted by NBC News in preparation for the news telecast about the microbe-CG-cancer cell breakthrough, NBC News reporter Roy Neal asked Dr. Rauscher if there was any scientific significance in finding a universal common denominator for all cancer cells. Dr. Rauscher replied, "This is what we have been looking for for years." When the video-taping was edited, Dr. Rauscher's statement was deleted due to the limited time element on the Segment Three section of the "NBC Nightly TV News." Of course, such a common denominator has been long sought, but after the NBC news broadcast nothing more developed from either Dr. Rauscher or the American Cancer Society. The news of the microbe-CG hormone breakthrough, moreover, had to come from the lay press rather than from an announcement by the cancer establishment. Why? Unfortunately, the Associated Press and the United Press International did not report upon the NBC News telecast, so nothing further appeared in the newspapers across the nation. NBC News is to be commended for having the courage to make the basic facts known on national television. Otherwise, no one would know or have the slightest notion that this breakthrough has even happened.

The *Montana Standard* newspaper in Butte, Montana carried the story in detail, however, and several other revealing articles in the months that followed the NBC News telecast, thanks to the fine efforts and reporting of staff writer, Rick Foote. Foote asked the AP if they would be interested in the story. He was informed that all cancer stories had to be cleared from the science editing department of the AP in New York. It would be interesting to see why this major story was not carried so that the rest of the nation could have read about it and followed the subsequent events. The city of Butte, Montana is probably the only area of the nation that has been fully informed as the story has unfolded. The Foote articles that appeared in the *Montana Standard* have been most helpful to the authors. By sending these news clips around to other newspapers, magazines, and representatives of TV news, they were able to provide facts to the media, although the media failed to inquire further or carry any additional stories of their own. This is a typical example of just how the news media is hypnotized by the cancer establishment. KXLF-TV in Butte and the Montana Television Network in Great Falls also provided some local and statewide coverage.

Like the National Cancer Institute, the American Cancer Society is often good for business. One good current example is the case of Interferon.

Discovered in 1957, Interferon is a substance produced in mammals when they are infected by a virus. The substance apparently stops the replication of viral genes. Since the Interferon is different for each species, all human Interferon must be extracted from human blood. Consequently, it is extremely expensive. Previous attempts to use the substance for cancer therapy have been described as "inconclusive."

However, in 1979 the ACS decided to spend 2.4 million dollars to purchase Interferon for use in treating cancer. The impression has been given that Interferon is something new, although it is not new at all.

Apparently this was one of the main topics at the annual ACS media meetings, since articles on Interferon have run recently in every publication except *Mad Magazine*. The American Cancer Society was, of course, the major consulting agency of the news media.

On January 16, 1980, Charles Weissman of the University of Zurich and Walter Gilbert from Harvard, both scientific advisors to Biogen, a European company specializing in recombinant DNA, announced in a press conference that the gene for

Interferon had been isolated and cloned, which meant that bacteria might well produce the substance in large quantities.

The effect of this announcement boosted the stock of Schering-Plough and International Nickel Corporation of Toronto (both share holders in Biogen) from 3⅝ to 37½ and from 2½ to 28⅞ in two days.[19]

In February 1980 the ACS announced that it would put another 3.4 million dollars into Interferon. Meanwhile, it has been estimated that American and European drug companies have already invested more than 100 million in research in hopes that Interferon will be a money maker like antibiotics.[10]

While everyone is concerned about how to manufacture Interferon artificially, Nobel Prize winner, Dr. Linus Pauling, has stated that large quantities of Vitamin C will increase the body's ability to produce Interferon *naturally*. In a national television interview on June 15, 1980, with Howard Ruff, on the program "Ruff House," Dr. Pauling candidly pointed out these millions of dollars as being a waste in expenditure when Vitamin C will do the job by itself when taken in proper quantities. But once the dollar mania enters the picture, scientific fact and the expertise of scientists like Dr. Pauling are brushed aside.

Preliminary reports on the use of Interferon as a potential treatment for cancer suggest that it is far from being an effective agent by any definition of the term and has serious side effects when administered to cancer patients.[4 11 14]

However, the net result has been a tremendous

amount of publicity for the American Cancer Society, which for 6.8 million dollars has received more than 10 million dollars in publicity.

Let us take a very close look at some of the clinical test results on Interferon thus far obtained. On May 28-31, 1980, the Seventy-First Annual Meeting of the American Association for Cancer Research was held in San Diego, California, in combination with the Sixteenth Annual Meeting of the American Society of Clinical Oncology, May 26-27, 1980.[14] At this prestigious meeting, clinical investigators from various research centers presented the initial clinical trial results of Interferon on some of the forms of cancer. These clinical trials were sponsored by the American Cancer Society. Although it is not possible to present all of the results in this book, here are a few examples from the official abstracts of the clinical report. In one study of 30 cases of multiple myeloma, a primary malignant tumor of the bone marrow, only 3 showed any disease regression. In another study of 5 cases of multiple myeloma, only one showed any response. Side effects, however, from the administration of Interferon were a decrease in the white blood cell count and a decrease in the normal amount of blood platelets needed for blood clotting. In some cases an increase and decrease in blood pressure also occurred. In a study of the effect of Interferon on breast cancer, 5 out of 16 patients gave a partial response. Again, a decrease in white blood cells resulted in one patient, and another developed pulmonary insufficiency. The results of Interferon on leukemia were similar. In a study of 7 patients only one showed any response. Three of these patients had adverse side effects of chills, fever, hypertension, labored breathing, and weakness. The most amazing part of these scientific abstracts is the conclusion reached that these results justify the effectiveness and further study of Interferon! For example, in the breast carcinoma study on the 5 out of 16 patients giving only partial response, the abstract states, "These findings confirm the therapeutic activity of HuLIF [human derived Interferon] in breast carcinoma." After reading the official reports, one might question how many patients might agree with this conclusion if given the choice of taking or not taking Interferon. The reader who wishes to pursue further the report on Interferon, should try to obtain a copy of these scientific reports. The dismal disappointment that Interferon is turning out to be is quite a different story than that presented by the news media to the public. The hypothesis has been set forth by the cancer powers that more purified Interferon is needed, at many more millions of dollars of expense, to further evaluate its activity.

Every year the American Cancer Society receives approximately 130 million dollars through donations. How much money does the ACS actually spend on research? From the advertising, one would think about 90 percent.

The truth is that research funds (highly touted by the ACS) total only about 28 *percent* of the total expenditures. Figures taken directly from the annual reports of the ACS show the following: In 1977, research totalled $35,651,933, or 29.7 percent.

This sounds like a lot of money until we realize that "supporting services" including management and fund raising take up about 22 percent of the budget. Further, *Penthouse* magazine states that the ACS has about 200 million dollars invested in various securities and in New York banks, making the organization a prime banking customer. Gary Null, the writer of the article, claims that some of the ACS board have connections with these banks.[13]

About 16 percent of the ACS budget goes into "public education," often, in effect, publicity for the American Cancer Society itself. Actually, the ACS shows a fairly typical pattern for fund-raising organizations. An article in the Columbus, Ohio, *Citizen Journal* for Friday, August 4, 1978, relates that in the state of Ohio, for example, the state division of the American Cancer Society, with a staff of some 200 persons (many of them making more than $20,000 a year), raised about 7.3 million dollars in 1977. The Ohio group spent less than $500,000 in research but more than 1.2 million dollars in overhead and fund-raising costs. It also sent some 2.7 million dollars to the national organization. Other organizations mentioned in the article were the Leukemia Society of America, which spent 40 percent of its income in fund-raising; and the Cancer Research Institute of New York, which spent $545,356 to raise $963,000! All of these organizations have salaried employees well above the poverty level.[17] A local cancer worker in Butte, Montana, known to one author, has complained about the small amount of money left in the community. He has also stated that the national ACS has pressured the local group to turn over money for a local cancer clinic established by a bequest.

In general, the vast amounts of money gathered through taxation and contributions have created a giant bureaucracy but have not made much headway against cancer. Research is not a primary activity of many private cancer groups in spite of their advertising or propaganda. What money is available is usually channeled into chemotherapy, carcinogens, viruses, and now the big Interferon extravaganza. Further, although research sponsored by these organizations themselves has identified a large number of carcinogenic chemicals, the "educational" material of the private cancer enterprise tends to blame the victim for *his* bad habits—smoking, sunbathing, and ignoring lumps.

The vast amounts of money spent in the name of cancer have created what James Watson (a Nobel laureate) has called

> "a new type of welfare system . . . more palatable because the recipients cannot solely sop up beer and watch TV, but instead will wear clean lab coats and look into cancer cells. Not being trained for the task, however, they are most unlikely to fathom the inner working of the cancer cell and in a ghoulish way will be forever assuring the continuation of their job description."[16]

The Zinder Report of 1974 said of the Special Virus Cancer Program, which had spent a half-billion dollars since 1964, that it had discovered nothing of value and had become a self-justifying organization. Those running the program, the report continued, formed a very narrow part of the scientific community and financed their own projects. Contracts were assigned for identical projects.[12]

Other reports have shown that scientists from universities and other research institutions who staff study section panels in many cases are receiving grants themselves from the ACS or the NCI for their own projects, or the institutions they represent are recipients of large grants for programs that are narrow and limited to the big three—viruses, carcinogens, chemotherapy. Meanwhile, the most promising area of research—immunology—has been funded very lightly, and valuable research proposals have been refused or assigned a low priority, as we have seen in the previous chapter. Dr. Michael Naughton, a top biochemist at the University of Colorado Medical Center, who was one of the first to work on CG in cancer cells, is a good example of a scientist who has been forced to discontinue his work for lack of money. Another is Dr. Vernon Stevens of Ohio State University School of Medicine, who for several years has done important work on the CG hormone, and is considered a foremost authority. His research has been funded entirely by the World Health Organization, to which he is a consultant.

Even Nobel laureates like Dr. Albert Szent-Gyorgyi and Dr. Linus Pauling receive no money from the NCI or ACS and depend upon public contributions to continue their research on the physics of cancer cells and the use of Vitamin C.

The picture of inequities, narrow vision, and

even provable corruption we have presented here is not meant to imply that either the NCI or the ACS is riddled with dishonest or indifferent people. However, the policing of large organizations and large amounts of money is beyond the capacity of organizations with few in-house scientists, who might give better direction to the way research money is spent. The real tragedy is that so much organization and money have resulted in so little.

Efforts to correct problems in cancer research are often little better than existing plans. For example, in 1978 Rep. Andrew McGuire (D–N.J.) introduced the Cancer Prevention Act (H.R. 10190).[8] This would put emphasis on prevention of cancer through the detection of carcinogens and the protection of workers and others from them. Instead of the big *three*—carcinogens, chemotherapy, and viruses—we would have the big *one*, carcinogens, being stressed. Again, in spite of the increasing promise of immunology for the prevention and treatment of cancer, we see the futile pursuit of the same old goals. Unless we are going to abandon our industrial society, the search for more carcinogens in the workplace and in the environment is an exercise in futility. Pouring money down the same rathole year after year may give the illusion that feverish efforts are being exerted to cure cancer, but actually a small segment of our society is benefiting lavishly from this folly.

The real problem is that most members of Congress are not scientists or men and women with much scientific training. Therefore, they must depend on "experts" for information on legislation concerning science and technology. Both Senator George McGovern and Senator Edward Kennedy have held hearings on cancer research with little result. Usually the National Cancer Institute and American Cancer Society official line prevails, and the status quo continues.

Certainly an exception to this is Senator John Melcher of Montana, who, in December 1979, introduced his bill, S. 2043, in the U.S. Senate entitled "The Animal Cancer Research Act." The manuscript of this book was used as the basis and springboard for Senator Melcher's bill. The Hearing Record is reproduced in this book (see appendix). This bill provides for animal studies in CG and cancer. In May of 1980 the bill passed the Senate unanimously and provided funding of 25 million dollars—more than what Senator Melcher originally requested. Senator Melcher's experience as a veterinarian gave him the scientific background to understand the biological research for the major breakthrough on cancer that it is.

In the House of Representatives the bill was recommended for passage after a hearing by the House Subcommittee on Department Investigations, Oversight, and Research of the Committee on Agriculture, Rep. E. (Kika) de la Garza, Texas, Chairman, and was passed by the House in the fall of 1980. President Carter then signed it into law. The House version of the bill provided that if money for this project is not appropriated, the funds will be taken from the NCI. The hearings and debate on this bill provided members of the Senate and the House with solid information on this important research based on the fact that cancer is a bacterial-related disease.

Much hope for change in the national cancer picture came with the appointment of Dr. Arthur C. Upton in July 1977 as director of the National Cancer Institute, since he had the support of the scientific community and of organized labor.* While it is true that Dr. Upton has moved away from the contract policy which led to abuses of funds in the past, he himself is an expert on radiation and carcinogenesis and is more interested in bioassay work than in basic cell research or immunology. In fact, researchers in contact with the authors have said that since Dr. Upton took over, less money seems to be available for areas like cell research and immunology in spite of an apparent increase in funds from Congress.

Throughout this book, we have been writing about research by excellent, highly recognized scientists, a very few of whom have been funded by either the NCI or the ACS.

*Note: Since this was written, Dr. Vincent T. DeVita, Jr. has become director of the NCI.

10

Summing Up

Important research dating back to 1902 on cancer-related bacteria has been ignored, suppressed, and forgotten. This research has resulted in perhaps the most important discovery in modern microbiology—the ability of certain cancer-related bacteria to naturally synthesize a human hormone: chorionic gonadotropin (CG) without genetic engineering. Discovered and announced by Dr. Virginia Livingston-Wheeler in 1974, this biochemical discovery is a scientific first and has been confirmed by expert microbiologists and biochemists in four highly regarded laboratories in different parts of the nation.

Other research has shown that CG is present on the surface of *every* cancer cell so far examined, that it is the *first universal biochemical characteristic* of cancer cells of all kinds, the first indication and confirmation that cancer is *one* disease regardless of its location or so-called "forms."

CG, with its strong negative electric charge, defeats the immune system, enabling cancer cells to invade and to metastasize.

The use of cancer-related bacteria which do synthesize a CG-like hormone, a practical preventive vaccine against CG synthesis and therefore against the development of cancer is virtually a certain development. This vaccine will come (along with more effective therapeutic agents based on CG destruction or modification) *soon* with adequate financial support, *eventually* with little or no support.

The directed research practices and other activities of the National Cancer Institute and of the American Cancer Society have been *scandalously* counterproductive in the conquest of cancer, in spite of the billions of dollars expended. The cancer establishment is closed to new approaches and ideas, thus creating a self-perpetuating system with no clear objective even remotely in sight.

Ultimately, because of the funding of research, the conquest of cancer may well be a matter of political decision and political action. Well-meaning members of Congress such as David Obey (D–Wisc.) and Andrew Maguire (D–N.J.) have at different times questioned the expensive cancer programs of the NCI, as have Senators George McGovern, Melcher, and Kennedy, and have brought to light important weaknesses in the cancer establishment.

Unfortunately, congressmen having to make decisions on scientific and technical matters rarely have the knowledge themselves to make intelligent appraisals and have to depend on experts—often people on their own staffs and people who have interests in the perpetuation of present practices or who are part of the agencies under scrutiny. Thus the cancer establishment tends to perpetuate its dogmas—which we and some eminent scientists consider folly—and nobody is the wiser. The cancer establishment has professional public relations people pumping out continual propaganda about how cancer is being conquered, although accurate statistics show this to be a lie. In a television interview in 1977, Dr. Arthur C. Upton, then Director of the NCI, admitted that the cure rate is basically no different for cancer than it was *30 years ago*. More specifically, the number of cancer cases is increasing each year, not declining.

What is needed is an informed public to ask Congress some real questions: Why have some five billion dollars been spent since 1973 with no gain at all on cancer? Is pouring money down the same rathole an effective answer?

The alternative to present practices is to turn once again to basic research on the biochemistry and physics of the cell—the normal cell and the malignantly transformed cell. The CG-microbe breakthrough has unquestionably opened this door wide. Why is every effort being made to stifle it?

As we have pointed out, the basic scientific work that we have summarized on these pages is startling and vastly important to human welfare. Yet it has taken place with virtually no support from official cancer research organizations. In fact, it has taken place practically *in spite* of the cancer establishment, with its emphasis on cancer centers and private industries.

Cancer will be conquered, as Dr. M. J. Scott

said, like smallpox and diphtheria, if the American people really want it to be conquered. But that day will not arrive if we go on in the same tired paths, the same old trails, when the most important road of all—prevention—has not been taken. Scientists like Drs. Acevedo and Slifkin, who have made important contributions to the study of tumors and cancer-associated bacteria, have been dependent upon small grants from individuals or foundations. For example, as a result of the NBC News presentation on Dr. Acevedo and Dr. Wheeler in 1977, Mr. Brooke Cadwallader, a businessman in Dallas, Texas, who saw the telecast, has given over $130,000 to both Acevedo and Wheeler. Dr. Acevedo, in particular, could not have continued his CG research had it not been for the contributions from Mr. Cadwallader. Moreover, this same philanthropist, at a cost of $24,000, sent a ten-page list of questions prepared by one of the authors (REN) by Telex to every member of Congress. The list of questions was prepared for Senator Warren Magnuson for use by the Senate Appropriations Committee in 1978. At that time the NCI convinced the Appropriations Committee that there was nothing to become excited about on this CG research. If, in fact, the research we have presented had depended upon the two main sources of funding—the National Cancer Institute and the American Cancer Society—it would never have been carried out.

Summing up, we can say that the funding of cancer research, particularly the tendency to target the research on areas like bioassay, chemotherapy, and viruses, has been a marked failure. Moreover, it has created what one can only call a vast "medical-industrial complex," feeding on millions of dollars and demanding more millions each year. When we consider the amounts of money spent on research, experimental treatment centers, chemicals, equipment like scanners (at least $750,000 each) and radiation devices, hospitalization, physician's fees, and cancer insurance, we are talking about hundreds of millions of dollars. No wonder biotechnology is thought to be the hottest investment area of the 1980s.

With all this money flowing, we cannot help ask the question: "Does anyone really want to conquer cancer?" To be sure, few researchers, few ethical physicians (most of whom are sincere, hard-working healers), radiologists, or executives of fund-raising organizations or drug or equipment manufacturing companies would consciously admit that they are afraid to see the end of cancer. Few would be as cynical as John Cairns, who states that the cure of lung cancer alone, which causes 101,000 deaths annually, would seriously imperil the social security system.[5] However, the failure of the cancer crusade, in spite of expenditures of over five billion dollars for research alone, suggests that this great flow of money may make many people *unconsciously* afraid that cancer will be conquered. For the day we see the end of cancer, the worst depression will hit the medical-industrial complex since Jonas Salk left the polio organization temporarily high and dry without a disease.

In view of the overall picture, who really wants to kill the golden goose?

11

Questions and Answers

Q. If CG is the common denominator of cancer, why was it not discovered long ago?

A. Detection of such substances in extremely small quantities at the level of the cell surface was not possible until the development of very recent technologies such as immunocytochemistry and radioimmunology.

Q. Why is there not more excitement in the scientific world about CG and cancer?

A. More scientists *are* working on CG now, but this is not an area that is heavily funded by either the NCI or the ACS. They have refused funding to scientists who wish to pursue it. We have written of the great conservatism of science. It might be added that although articles have appeared in significant journals, the great number of journals and the fact that many scientists do not read some articles in journals they receive means that the *significance* of this particular research has not appeared to a great number of researchers. It is not, after all, part of the great triad of carcinogens, chemotherapy, and virus research.

Q. Has the NCI funded *any* CG hormone research?

A. In answer to Congressional inquiries, in 1978, representatives boasted that they have put out approximately $300,000 in this area (out of 900 million plus). Most of this research has not been on CG at the cellular level, however. This is a critical point to understand in order to distinguish between meticulous research and gross, sloppy research even though it may be on the same target. Further, the CG-producing cancer-related bacteria are being totally ignored, in spite of their importance to the future of a cancer vaccine. Compare the statements of representatives of the Department of Agriculture in the Senate Subcommittee Hearing reprinted in the appendix.

Q. Does a bacterial vaccine against cancer or early diagnosis using CG have anything to do with "unproven cures" (ACS terminology) like Laetrile or Krebiozen?

A. Absolutely not. There is no comparison. The CG-like hormone is part of the transformation process by which a normal cell becomes a malignant cell. The emphasis here is on *prevention*, from allowing the malignant process from occurring in the first place. Although as we have stated, possible effective therapies might be developed in anti-CG agents.

Laetrile, which is made from apricot pits and which has been around since the 1920s is, as we have stated, a form of chemotherapy. The active ingredient in Laetrile is supposed to release hydrogen cyanide at the site of cancer cells. The biochemistry has nothing to do with CG.

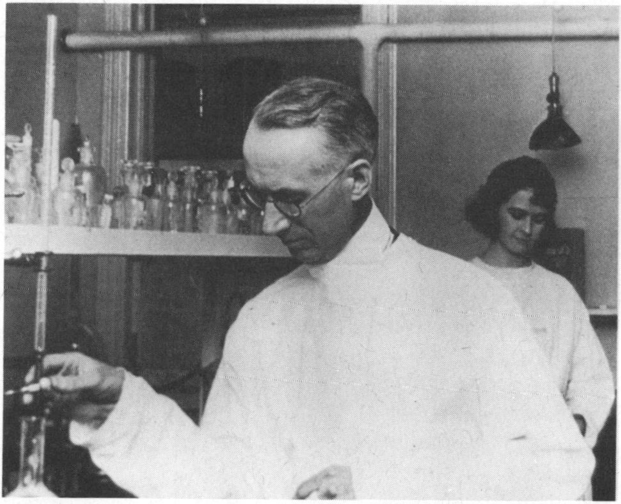

Dr. Michael J. Scott in the laboratory about 1924. In the background is Scott's sister, Mary, who assisted him.

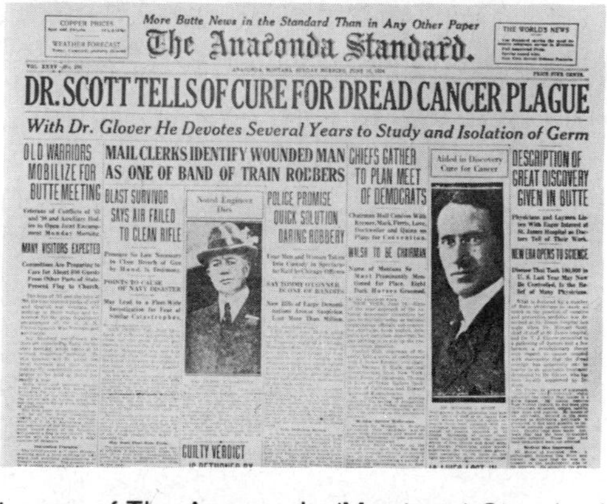

More Butte News in the Standard Than in Any Other Paper

The Anaconda Standard.

COPPER PRICES

WEATHER FORECAST

THE WORLD'S NEWS

DR. SCOTT TELLS OF CURE FOR DREAD CANCER PLAGUE

With Dr. Glover He Devotes Several Years to Study and Isolation of Germ

OLD WARRIORS MOBILIZE FOR BUTTE MEETING

MANY VISITORS EXPECTED

MAIL CLERKS IDENTIFY WOUNDED MAN AS ONE OF BAND OF TRAIN ROBBERS

BLAST SURVIVOR SAYS AIR FAILED TO CLEAN RIFLE

POINTS TO CAUSE OF NAVY DISASTER

Noted Engineer Dies

POLICE PROMISE QUICK SOLUTION DARING ROBBERY

CHIEFS GATHER TO PLAN MEET OF DEMOCRATS

WALSH TO BE CHAIRMAN

Aided in Discovery Cure for Cancer

DESCRIPTION OF GREAT DISCOVERY GIVEN IN BUTTE

NEW ERA OPENS TO SCIENCE

GUILTY VERDICT

Front page of The Anaconda (Montana) Standard, *June 15, 1924, showing Scott's announcement of cancer bacteria—antiserum discovery.*

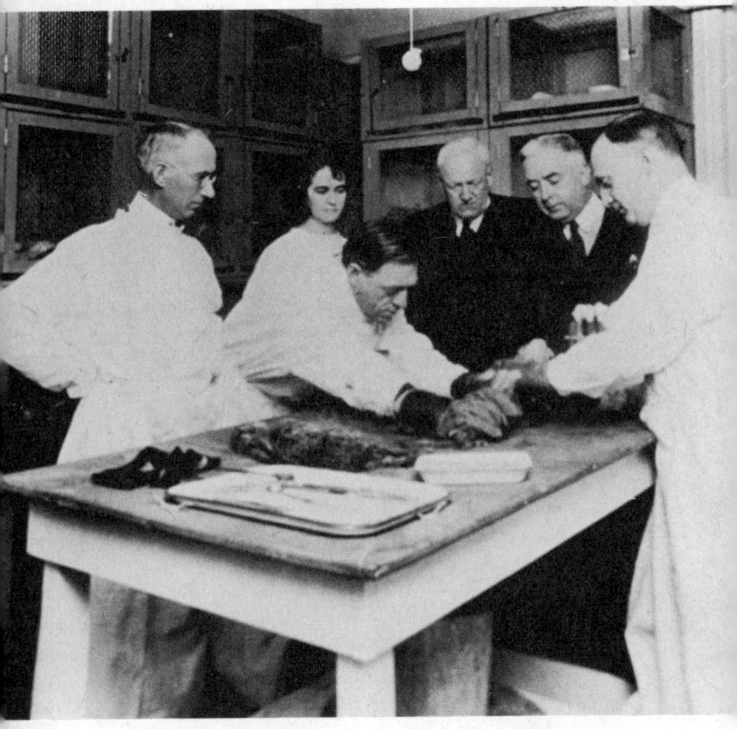

In Dr. Glover's laboratory in New York City, about 1924. From left to right, Dr. Michael J. Scott, Thomas J. Deaken, Mary Scott, unknown, Dr. Thomas J. Glover, unknown.

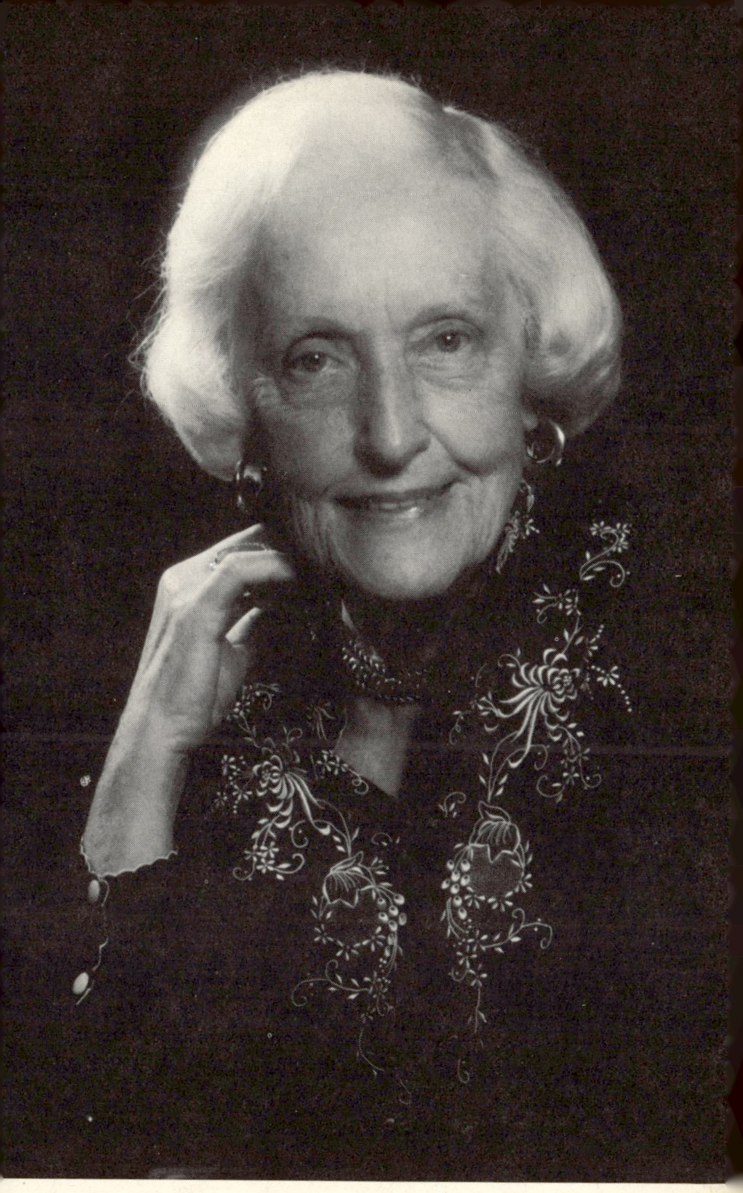

Virginia Livingston-Wheeler, M.D., San Diego, California.

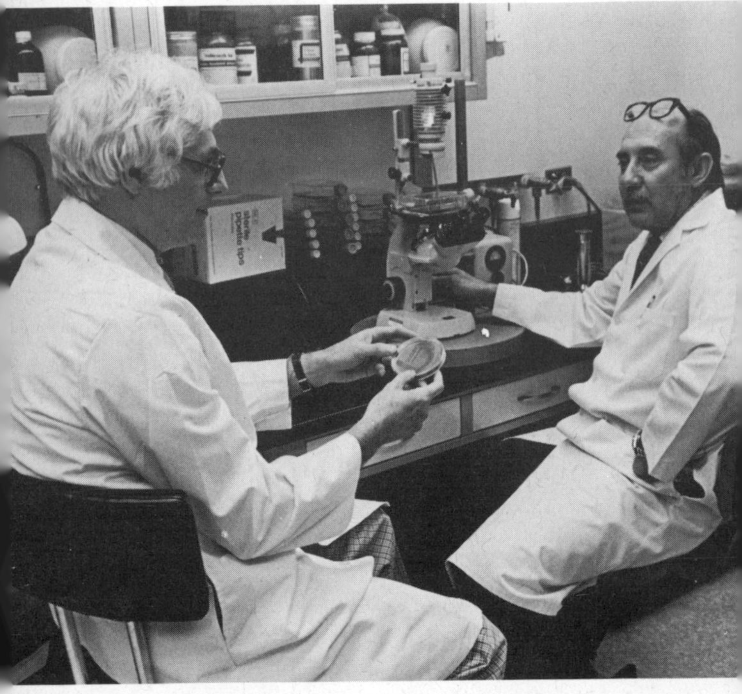

Malcolm Slifkin, Ph.D., Head, Section of Microbiology—Immunology, and Herman F. Acevedo, Ph.D., Senior Scientist, Head, Section of Research, Department of Laboratory Medicine, Allegheny General Hospital, Pittsburgh, Pennsylvania.

Q. Why have we never read in popular magazines about CG or heard about it on TV as we have about Interferon?

A. Most of the scientific writers for mass media depend upon the National Cancer Institute and to a greater extent on the American Cancer Society's annual meetings for science writers. At these meetings they accept and publish what is handed to them. Few have the time or the incentive to investigate the claims or read a lot of journal material in hope of finding something missed by the authorities they have come to depend on. It becomes a very comfortable "flow with the tide" situation. They also are rewarded for publishing articles that put out the American Cancer Society "line." In general, the media have been the least likely people in the United States to "rock the boat," with the exception of the excellent NBC News presentation in 1977 on CG and CG-producing bacteria and the possibility of a universal cancer vaccine. The rest of the news media ignored the NBC News presentation, which in light of the latest confirmatory results on the cancer cells and bacterial microbes, becomes all the more significant.

Q. Why doesn't my doctor know about this work on CG and CG-producing bacteria?

A. Doctors depend upon journal articles (when they get time to read journals in their busy lives). Most of what they read is on the level of applied, rather than basic research, which means the use of toxic, dangerous chemicals under the name of chemotherapy. And unless they have really passionate interest in research, they get most of their information on what is "significant" in cancer research from the mass media, who have previously received it from the American Cancer Society, the NCI, or other entrenched segments of the cancer establishment.

Q. Have scientists ever tried to produce cancer in animals by injecting them with live bacteria from cancer patients?

A. Yes, many times, usually unsuccessfully. This has given much ammunition to the cancer establishment because the injection of bacteria has not necessarily produced animal tumors. However, in view of the latest research, it is not likely that injection of bacteria *would* produce cancer. Transformation of the cells is a slow, complex process involving DNA transfer or exchange and possibly cell injury. However, as we have stated in chapter four, the workers at the NIH laboratories in the 1930s *did* succeed in producing cancer in animals from bacteria derived from human cancer patients.

The production of malignant tumors or lesions with the microbes is no longer a valid argument. The microbe responsible for leprosy has *never* produced the disease in an animal, and if the microbe is injected into a human being, it virtually never causes the disease to appear. Still, when *conditions* are right, leprosy is a contagious disease. Although the disease does not result when the microbe is injected into experimental animals or human beings, no one disputes the fact that leprosy is a bacteria-caused disease.

Our concern here is not so much whether or not bacteria are in some way responsible for cancer (we suspect they are), but the promise of these bacteria in the preparation of a vaccine.

Q. Are the bacterial microbes extracted from cancer patients and found to be producing a CG-like hormone pathogenic, that is, do they have the ability to produce disease?

A. Usually not. As a matter of fact, Dr. Acevedo has described these various bacteria as the common "Joe Smiths" of the bacteria world. One such bacterium is *E. coli*, commonly found in the human intestine. Some strains, all taken from cancer patients, produce the CG-like hormone. The idea that a bacteria connected with cancer must be harmful in the same way as the bacteria that cause pneumonia or Legionnaire's Disease is a false one.

Q. You are saying that the scientific basis for a vaccine is here and ready to be applied. How can all of this be so simple when we have been led to believe that cancer is a deeply complicated disease requiring hundreds of millions of dollars to solve?

A. To many scientists, cancer is a complicated disease having many forms and manifestations with the resulting belief that it is not one but hundreds of diseases. This is why so much money has been spent in unfruitful directions, because no one has believed that any "magic bullet" could be found for cancer any more than for the common cold, which is also thought by some scientists to be many "diseases" also.

However, the discovery of a universal antigen (CG) on all cancer cells, regardless of location or the production of other substances (cancer cells are regular chemical factories) means that cancer is *one* disease with many manifestations or *forms.* One characteristic, particularly one which functions as a protection of the cancer cell against the body's immune defenses, is enough to define cancer and to see that at least so far as prevention is concerned, the "magic bullet" is on the way. The research at such great expense on carcinogens, chemotherapy, and viruses will for the most part go down in history as a form of human folly, blended well with directions that have brought self-perpetuation and financial gain to some. One cannot say scientific folly, since the science has often been excellent, just aimed at the wrong target.

Q. What about the use of Vitamin C in cancer therapy?

A. Ascorbate (Vitamin C) has been recommended in the prevention and treatment of cancer by Dr. Linus Pauling and associates. According to their publications, Vitamin C is important in two ways: (1) strengthening collagen in the intercellular material, (2) stimulating the immune system, including the formation of Interferon. Recent tests of Vitamin C at Mayo Clinic were reviewed negatively, but Pauling says that chemotherapy treatment before the use of Vitamin C makes the immune stimulation virtually useless. This is promising research. Vitamin C and other substances may very well supplement the vaccine in keeping the immune system active.

Q. Is cancer caused by viruses?

A. In the sense that viruses, like other carcinogens, can "cause" cancer, the answer can be considered a qualified yes. Vaccines prepared against viruses as a prevention or treatment for human cancer have been a failure, although literally hundreds of millions of dollars have been spent to develop a viral vaccine. Now that the connection between CG-producing bacteria and cancer cells has been demonstrated, it becomes clear why this vast expenditure has been a failure.

Q. Is cancer hereditary?

A. Statistically it might be so described. However, so little is known about the precise mechanisms of malignant transformation that we may well be looking at defects in the immune system, which may be genetically transmitted. Some forms of cancer in infants seem certainly to be due to genetic malfunction. This question may eventually be solved by geneticists but it has no bearing on whether or not we can have a universal preventive vaccine for cancer. The main point to remember is that no matter how the cancer is induced, or promoted, whether it be due to carcinogens, viruses, or hereditary factors, the CG-synthesis seems to be the basic biochemical process of every cancer cell. To vaccinate against the CG-producing bacterial microbes which can be freely isolated from any cancer patient is the main goal.

Q. How has the cancer establishment gotten by for so many decades leading everyone down a blind alley on cancer by blaming everything from smoking to asbestos as being "causes" of cancer when these are only predisposing causes to the basic bacterial-CG-cancer cell process?

A. Only a full Congressional investigation can bring some answers to this and many other questions that the people of this nation will ask. Certainly there can be no excuses for not knowing of the discovery since all details of the CG discovery have appeared in top medical journals as well as on the NBC Nightly TV News. Why it was ignored should be the first question of paramount importance.

REFERENCES

INTRODUCTION

1. U.S. Chamber of Commerce, Bureau of the Census. *Historical Statistics of the United States*. Washington, D.C.: Government Printing Office, 1975.

2. Rettig, Richard. *Cancer Crusade*. Princeton, N.J.: Princeton University Press, 1975.

Chapter One

1. *Anaconda Standard*. 35:1, June 15, 1924.

2. Boesch, Mark. *The Long Search for the Truth About Cancer*. New York: G. P. Putnam, 1960. (Most of the information on Scott is based on personal interviews by REN with Scott.)

3. Scott, Michael. "Clinical Experiences with Carcinoma Antitoxin." *Irish Journal of Cancer*, 3 (9): 1-6, 1926.

4. Scott, Michael. "The Parasitic Origin of Carcinoma: Arguments in Favor of the Parasitic Etiology of Cancer." *Northwest Medicine*, April 1925.

5. Young, James. "A New Outlook on Cancer: Irritation and Infection." *British Medical Journal*, 3341: 60, 1925.

Chapter Two

1. American Cancer Society: *American Cancer Society Annual Report*. New York: ACS, 1977.

2. Koestler, Arthur. *The Ghost in the Machine*. New York: MacMillan, 1968.

Chapter Three

1. Cameron, Ewan, Linus Pauling. *Cancer and Vitamin C*. Menlo Park, CA: Linus Pauling Institute of Science and Medicine, 1979.

2. Moss, Ralph. *The Cancer Syndrome*. New York: Grove Press, 1980.

3. McCann, Jean. "What Cancer Experts Do to Keep from Getting Cancer." *Good Housekeeping* (May, 1970), 190-191.

Chapter Four

1. Alexander-Jackson, Eleanor. "A New Differential Stain Technique for the Study of *M. Tuberculosis* in Tissues and Body Fluids." *Science* 99: 307-308, 1944.

2. Boesch, Mark. *The Long Search for the Truth About Cancer*. New York: G.P. Putnam, 1960.

3. Cantwell, Alan R. Jr., Dan W. Kelso. "Acid-Fast

Bacteria in Scleroderma and Morphea." *Arch Derm.* *104*: 21-25, 1971.

4. Clark, George A. *Successful Culturing of Glover's Cancer Organism and Development of Metastasizing Tumors in Animals Produced by Cultures from Human Malignancy.* Pittsburgh: Privately Printed, 1953.

5. Crofton, W. M. *The True Nature of Viruses.* London: Staples Press, Ltd., 1936.

6. Delmotte, N. and L. Van Der Mieren. "Recherches bacteriologiques et histologogiques concernant la sclerodermie.". *Dermatologica.* 107 (3): 117-182, 1953.

7. Fonti, Clara. *Etiopatogenese del Cancro.* Milano-Varese: Inst. Editoriale Cisalpino, A. Nicola & Co., 1958.

8. Gerlach, Franz. *Krebs und obligater Pilzparasitismus.* Wein: Urban u. Schwarzenberg, 1948.

9. Glover, T. J., J. L. Engle. *Studies in Malignancy.* New York: Murdock Foundation, 1938.

10. Glover, T. J., J. E. White. *The Treatment of Cancer in Man.* New York: Murdock Foundation, 1940.

11. Livingston, Afton Munk, Virginia Wuerthele-Caspe Livingston (Wheeler), Eleanor Alexander-Jackson, Gerhard Wolter. "Toxic Fractions Obtained from Tumor Isolates and Related Clinical Implications." *Annals of the New York Academy of Sciences,* 174: 675-689, 1970.

12. Natenberg, Maurice. *The Cancer Blackout.* Chicago: Regent House, 1959.

13. Rose, S. J., Virginia Wuerthele-Caspe (Wheeler), Roy M. Allen. "The Presence of Consistently Recurring Invasive Mycobacterial Forms in Tumor Cells." *Newark Medical Women's Journal,* August 1947.

14. Seibert, Florence, J. Kierking, R. L. Davis. "Bacterial Isolates from Tumors: One Organism or Many?" *International. Research. Communications. Systems*, March 1973.

15. (Wheeler) Wuerthele-Caspe Livingston, Eleanor Alexander-Jackson. "An Experimental Biologic Approach to the Treatment of Neoplastic Disease." *Journal of the American Women's Association*, 20 (8): 858-866, 1965.

16. Wheeler, Virginia (Wuerthele-Caspe Livingston). *Cancer: A New Breakthrough.* San Diego: Production House, 1972.

17. (Wheeler) Wuerthele-Caspe (Livingston), Virginia, E. Alexander-Jackson, J. A. Anderson, J. Hillier, L. W. Smith. "Cultural Properties and Pathogenicity of Certain Microorganisms Obtained from Various Proliferative and Neoplastic Diseases." *American Journal of Medical Sciences*, 220: 628-646, 1950.

18. (Wheeler) Wuerthele-Caspe Livingston, A. M. Livingston. "Demonstration of Progenitor Cryptocides in the Blood of Patients with Collagen and Neoplastic Diseases." *Transactions of the New York Academy of Sciences*, 28: 433-453, 1972.

19. (Wheeler) Wuerthele-Caspe (Livingston), Virginia, Eva Brodkin, Camille Mermod. "Etiology of Scleroderma, a Preliminary Report." *Journal of the Medical Society of New Jersey*, 44(7): 256, 1947.

20. (Wheeler) Wuerthele-Caspe (Livingston), Virginia, E. Alexander-Jackson, M. Gregory, L. W. Smith, I.C. Diller, Z. Manowski. "Intercellular Acid-Fast Microorganism Isolated from Two Cases of Heptolenticular Degeneration." *Journal of the American Medical Women's Association*, 11:120-129, 1956.

21. (Wheeler) Wuerthele-Caspe (Livingston), Vir-

ginia. "Microbiology of Cancer, Neoplastic Infection in Man and Animals." *Atti del VI Congresso Internazionale di Microbiologia*, 6 (sez. XVII): 3-9, 1953.

22. (Wheeler) Wuerthele-Caspe (Livingston), Virginia. "Microorganisms Associated with Neoplasms." *New York Microscopical Society Bulletin*, 2: 2-31, 1948.

23. (Wheeler) Wuerthele-Caspe (Livingston), Virginia, E. Alexander-Jackson, Lawrence Weld Smith. "Some Aspects of the Microbiology of Cancer." *Journal of the American Medical Women's Association*, 8(1): 7-12, 1953.

24. (Wheeler) Wuerthele-Caspe (Livingston), Virginia, Eleanor Alexander-Jackson. "A Specific Type of Organism Cultivated from Malignancy: Bacteriology and Proposed Classification." *Annals of the New York Academy of Sciences*, 174: 636-654, 1970.

25. White, John E. "Report of 100 Pathologically Proven Cases of Malignancy Treated by a Specific Antiserum." In Virginia Livingston Wheeler and Owen Webster Wheeler. *The Microbiology of Cancer*. San Diego: Livingston-Wheeler Clinic, 1977.

Chapter Five

1. Acevedo, H. F., M. Slifkin, G. R. Pouchet, M. Rakhshan. "Identification of the B-subunit of Choriogonadotropin (CG) in Human Spermatozoa" in *The Testis in Normal and Infertile Men*, ed. P. Troen and H. R. Nankin. New York: Raven Press, 1977, pp. 185-192.

2. Acevedo, H. F., M. Slifkin, M. Pardo, G. R. Pouchet, M. Rakhshan. "Human Chorionic Gonado-

tropin in Cancer Cells. I. Identification in *in vitro* and *in vivo* Cancer-Cell Systems. In *Detection and Prevention of Cancer,* Part 2, Vol. I. ed. H. E. Nieburg. New York: Marcel Dekker, Inc. 1978, pp. 957-963.

3. Acevedo, H. F., M. Slifkin, G. R. Pouchet, M. Pardo. "Immunohistochemical Localization of a Choriogonadotropin-like Protein in Bacteria Isolated from Cancer Patients." *Cancer,* 41: 1217-229, 1978.

4. Acevedo, H. F., M. Slifkin, G. R. Pouchet-Melvin, E. A. Campbell-Acevedo. "Choriogonadotropin-like Antigen in the Anaerobic Bacterium, *Eubacterium lentum,* Isolated from Rectal Tumor." *Infection and Immunity,* 24: 920-924, 1979.

5. Adejuwon, Christopher, S. J. Segal, S. Mitsudo. "Protease Inhibitor Abolishes the Apparent hCG-like immunactivity in Human Tissues." Program of the Endocrine Society 61st Annual Meeting, June 1979, Abst. 954.

6. Asch, R. H., E. O. Fernandez, C. J. Pauerstein. "Immunodetection of hCG-like Substance in Human Sperm." *Fertility and Sterility,* 28: 1258-1262, 1977.

7. August, Charles, S. Cox, M. Naughton. "Resistance of Cultured Choriocarcinoma Cells to Cell-mediated Cytotoxicity of Mitogen-Activated Lymphocytes." *Journal of Clinical Investigations,* 63: 428-436, 1979.

8. Beard, J. "Embryological Aspects and Etiology of Cancer." *Lancet,* 1: 1758, 1902.

9. Beck, J. S., I. B. Porteous, J. L. Ullyot. "Gonadotropin-secreting Bronchial Carcinoma: Aberrant Endocrine Activity or Trophoblastic Differentiation?" *Journal of Pathology,* 101: 59-62, 1970.

10. Braunstein, G. D., J. L. Vaitukaitis, P. P. Carone, G. T. Ross. "Ectopic Production of Human Chorionic

Gonadotropin by Neoplasms.". *Annals. of. Internal Medicine*, 78: 39-45, 1973.

11. Braunstein, G. D., V. K. Kamdar, J. Kanabus, J. Rasor. "Properties of Human Chorionic Gonadotropin Produced *in vitro* by Ovarian Carcinoma Cells." *Journal of Clinical Endocrinology and Metabolism*, 47: 326-332, 1978.

12. Chou, Janice Y., S. S. Want, J. C. Robinson. "Regulation of the Synthesis of Human Chorionic Gonadotropin by 5-Bromo 2′-deoxyuridine and Dibutyrl Cyclic AMP in Trophoblastic and Nontrophoblastic Tumor Cells." *Journal of Clinical Endocrinology and Metabolism*, 47: 46-51, 1978.

13. Cohen, H., A. Strampp. "Bacterial Synthesis of Substances Similar to Human Chorionic Gonadotropin." *Proceedings of the Society of Experimental Biology and Medicine*, 152: 408-410, 1976.

14. Comings, David. "Lymphocyte Transformation in Response to Phytohemagluttinin During and Following a Pregnancy." *American Journal of Obstetrics and Gynecology*, 97: 213-217, 1967.

15. Defendi, V. G. Gasic. "Surface Mucopolysaccharides of Polyoma Virus Transformed Cells." *Journal of Cell Composition Physiology*, 62: 23-26, 1963.

16. Domingue, Gerald, Bruce Turner and Jorgen U. Schlegel, 1974. "Cell-wall Deficient Bacterial Variants in Kidney Tissue. Detection by Immunofluorescence." *Urology*, 3: 288.

17. Domingue, Gerald J., H. B. Woody, K. B. Farris, and J. U. Schlegel. "Demonstration of Bacterial Variants in Urinary Casts and Renal Epithelial Cells," 1979. *Archives of Internal Medicine*, 139: 1355.

18. Domingue, Gerald J., "Filterable Cell-

Associated Cryptic Bacterial Forms in Immunologic Renal Diseases." *Urological Survey*, 30: 1, 1980.

19. Domingue, Gerald, Keith Lloyd, and J. U. Schlegel, 1974. "*In Vitro* Phagocytosis of Transitional Phase Bacterial Variants Utilizing Autoradiography." *Proceedings of the Society for Experimental Biology and Medicine.* 146: 635.

20. Domingue, Gerald J., Jorgen U. Schlegel, and Hannah B. Woody, "Naked Bacteria in Human Blood," 1976. A Novel Concept for Etiology of Certain Kidney Diseases. *Microbia*, 2: 3.

21. Domingue, Gerald J., J. U. Schlegel, P. M. Heidger, Jr., and Melanie Ehrlich, 1976. In L-forms Protoplasts and Spheroplasts J. Roux, Ed. Novel Bacterial Structures in Human Blood: Cultural Isolation, Ultrastructural and Biochemical Evaluation.. *INSERM*, 21: 279.

22. Domingue, Gerald J. and Jorgen U. Schlegel, 1977. "Novel Bacterial Structures in Human Blood I. Cultural Isolation." *Infection and Immunity*, 15: 621.

23. Domingue, Gerald J. and Jorgen U. Schlegel, 1978. "Novel Bacterial Structures in Human Blood II. Bacterial Variants as Etiologic Agents in Idiopathic Hematuria." *Journal of Urology*, 120: 708.

24. Domingue, Gerald J. and Jorgen U. Schlegel, 1970. The Possible Role of Microbial L-forms in Pyelonephritis. *Journal of Urology*, 104: 790.

25. Fauve, Robert M., B. Hevin, H. Jacob, J. Gaillard, F. Jacob. "Antiinflammatory Effects of Murine Malignant Cells." *Proceedings of the National Academy of Science*, 71: 4052-4056, 1974.

26. Fontain, Yves-Alain, E. Burzawa-Gerard. "Esquisse de L'Evolution des Hormones Gonadotropes et

Thyreotropes des Vertebres." *General and Comparative Endocrinology*, 32: 341-347, 1977.

27. Ghosh, Ninaik, A. Rukenstein, R. P. Cox. "Induction of Human Choriogonadotropin in HeLa-Cell Cultures by Aliphatic Monocarboxylates and Inhibition of Deoxyribonucleic Acid Synthesis." *Biochemical Journal*, 166: 265-274, 1977.

28. Green, Mary T., Paul M. Heidger, Jr., and Gerald Domingue, 1974. "Demonstration of the Phenomena of Microbial Persistence and Reversion with Bacterial L-forms in Human Embryonic Kidney Cells." *Infection and Immunity*, 10: 889.

29. Green, Mary T., Paul M. Heidger, Jr., and Gerald Domingue, 1974. "A Proposed Life Cycle for a Relatively Stable L-Phase Variant of *Streptococcus faecalis*." *Infection and Immunity*, 10: 915.

30. Malkin, A., J. A. Kellen, A. Kolin, R. Cameron, E. Faber. "The Immunohistochemical Detection of Chorionic Gonadotropin in Experimental Rat Hepatomas." *Scandinavian Journal of Immunology*, 8 (sup. 8): 603-607, 1978.

31. Maruo, T., H. Cohen, S. J. Segal, and S. S. Koide. "Production of Choriogonadotropin-like Factor by a Microorganism." *Proc. Natl. Acad. Sci. USA*, 76: 6622, 1979.

32. McManus, L. M., M. A. Naughton, Q. Martinez-Hernandez. "Human Chorionic Gonadotropin in Human Neoplastic Cells.". *Cancer. Research*, 36: 3476-3481, 1976.

33. Muggia, F. M., S. W. Rosen, B. D. Weintraub, H. H. Hansen. "Ectopic Placental Proteins in Nontrophoblastic Tumors: Serial Measurements Following Chemotherapy." *Cancer* 36: 1327-1337, 1976.

34. Pattillo, Roland A., M. R. Facog, M. R. Shalaby, R. O. Hussa, O. P. Bahl, R. F. Mattingly. "Effect of Crude and Purified hCG on Lymphocyte Blastogenesis." *Obstetrics and Gynecology*, 47: 557-561, 1976.

35. Pattillo, Roland A. "Trophoblastic Cancers: Chorionic Gonadotropin Hormone Production, Antigenic Expression, and Trophoblastic Redifferentiation in Multiple Forms of Malignancy." *Pathology Annual*. New York: Appleton Century Crofts, 1973.

36. Quiones, Jose, G. Mizejewski, W. H. Beierwaltes. "Choriocarcinoma Scanning Using Radiolabeled Antibody to Chorionic Gonadotropin." *Journal of Nuclear Medicine*, 12: 69-72, 1970.

37. Ross, Griff. "Clinical Relevance of Research in the Structure of Human Chorionic Gonadotropin." *American Journal of Obstetrics and Gynecology*, 29: 795-808, 1977.

38. Schlegal-Haueter, Susanna, E., J. C. Robinson, Janice Y. Chou. "Characterization of Human Chorionic Gonadotropin Synthesized by Human Cell Lines." Program of the Endocrine Society 60th Annual Meeting, June 1978, Abst. 43.

39. Segal, Sheldon. "Immunological Methods to Prevent Pregnancy: An Editorial Comment." *Contraception*, 13: 124-127, 1976.

40. Simmons, Richard, V. Cruse, D. G. McKay. "The Immunological Problem of Pregnancy.". *American Journal of Obstetrics and Gynecology*, 97: 218-230, 1967.

41. Slifkin, M., H. F. Acevedo, M. Pardo, G. R. Pouchet, M. Rakhshan. "Human Chorionic Gonadotropin in Cancer Cells, II. Ultra-structural Localization." *In Detection and Prevention of Cancer*, Part 2,

Vol. I, ed. H. E. Nieburgs. New York: Marcel Dekker, 1978, pp. 965-979.

42. Slifkin, M., M. Pardo, G. R. Pouchet-Melvin, H. F. Acevedo. "Immuno-electron Microscopic Localization of a Chorio-gonadotropin-like Antigen in Cancer-Associated Bacteria." *Oncology*, 36: 208-210, 1979.

43. Van Beek, W. P., L. A. Smets, P. Emmelot. "Changed Surface Glycoprotein as a Marker of Malignancy in Human Leukemic Cells.". *Nature*, 253: 457-460, 1975.

44. (Wheeler) Wuerthele-Caspe Livingston, Virginia, A. M. Livingston. "Some Cultural, Immunological, and Biochemical Properties of Progenitor Cryptocides." *Transactions of the New York Academy of Sciences*, 36: 569-582, 1974.

45. Whyte, A., Y. W. Loke, "Increased Sialylation of Surface Glycopeptides of Human Trophoblast Compared with Fetal Cells from the Same Conceptus." *Journal of Experimental Medicine*, 148: 1087-1092, 1978.

Chapter Six

1. Papers from Scientists of the All India Institute of Medical Sciences, *Contraception*, 13: 131-268, 1976.

2. Seibert, Florence B., R. L. Davis. "Delay in Tumor Development Induced with a Bacterial Vaccine." *Journal of the Reticuloendothelial Society*, 21: 279-282, 1977.

3. Stevens, Vernon C. "Immunization of Female Baboons with Hapten-Coupled Gonadotropins." *Obstetrics and Gynecology*, 42: 496-506, 1973.

4. Talwar, G. P., N. C. Sharma, S. K. Dubey, M.

Salahuddin, C. Das, S. Romarishan, S. Kumar, V. Hingorani. "Iso-immunization against Human Chorionic Gonadotropin with Conjugates of Processed B-subunit of the Hormone and Tetanus Toxoid." *Proceedings of the National Academy of Sciences,* USA, 73: 218-222, 1976.

5. Maruo, Takesi, S. J. Segal, S. S. Koide. "Studies on the Apparent Human Chorionic Gonadotropin-like Factor in the Crab *Ovalipes ocellatus.*" *Endocrinology,* 104: 932-939, 1979.

6. Wass, M., K. McCann, K. D. Bagshawe. "Isolation of Antibodies to hCG/LH from Human Sera." *Nature,* 274: 368-370, 1978.

Chapter Seven

1. Goldenberg, E. E. Kim, F. H. DeLand, J. R. van Nagell, Jr., N. Javadpour. "Clinical Radioimmunodetection of Cancer with Radioactive Antibodies to Human Chorionic Gonadotropin." *Science,* 208:1284-1286, 1980.

2. Kellen, J. A., A. Kolin, J. A. Teodroczyk, A. Malkin. "Effect of Pre-Treatment with Antisera against Choriogonadotropin on the Metastic Potential of a Rat Adenocarcinoma EORTO Report on Metastasis, *in press.*

3. Wade, Nicholas. "Hybridomas: A Potent New Biotechnology." *Science,* 208: 692-693, 1980.

4. *Wall Street Journal,* October 24, 1978, 1.

Chapter Eight

1. Bronowski, Jacob. *The Ascent of Man.* Boston: Little-Brown, 1973.

2. Carter, Richard. *Breakthrough: The Saga of Jonas Salk.* New York: Trident Press, 1966.

3. Cohan, Liza Z. "Papanicolaou: The Gentle Giant." *Lab. World,* March 1979, 25-30.

4. Cole, Stephen, Leonard C. Rubin, Jonathan R. Cole. "Peer Review and the Support of Science." *Scientific American,* 237: 34-41, 1977.

5. Kuhn, Thomas. *The Structure of Scientific Revolutions.* Chicago: University of Chicago Press, 1970.

6. Osler, William. *A Way of Life.* London: Oxford University Press, 1951. From *A Way of Life and Other Selected Writings of William Osler,* by permission of Oxford University Press.

7. "Penicillin.". *Encyclopaedia. Britannica,* 17: 464-466, 1956.

8. Price, Lucian. *Dialogues With Alfred North Whitehead.* Boston: Little-Brown, 1954.

9. "Semmelweiss." *Encyclopaedia Britannica,* 20: 318, 1956.

Chapter Nine

1. American Cancer Society, *Annual Report,* 1977. New York: American Cancer Society, 1977.

2. American Cancer Society. *Annual Report,* 1978. New York: American Cancer Society, 1978.

3. American Cancer Society. *Annual Report*, 1979. New York: American Cancer Society, 1979.

4. Bordon, E., T. Dao, J. Holland, J. Gutterman, T. Merrigan. "Interferon in Recurrent Breast Carcinoma: Preliminary Report of the American Cancer Society Clinical Trials Program." Abstract #750, *Proceedings*, Seventy-First Meeting of the American Association for Cancer Research/Sixteenth Annual Meeting of the American Society of Clinical Oncology, 1980.

5. Cairns, John. *Cancer, Science, and Society*. San Francisco: W. H. Freeman, 1978.

6. Comptroller General of the United States. *Need To Improve Administration of a Carcinogen Testing and Carcinogenesis Research Contract*. Washington: United States General Accounting Office, 1978.

7. Comptroller General of the United States. *Review of the Procurement of 5-Fluorodeoxyudridine, An Experimental Cancer Drug by National Institutes of Health, Education, and Welfare*. Washington: United States General Accounting Office, 1960.

8. Epstein, Samuel S. *The Politics of Cancer*. San Francisco: Sierra Books, 1978.

9. Goddard, James L. "The Medical Business." *Scientific American*: 229 (Sept. 1973), 161-168.

10. "Industry Readies for Interferon Market." *Science*, 207, 1326, 1980.

11. Krown, S. E., M. B. Stoopler, S. Cunningham-Rundles, H. F. Oettgen. "Phase II Trial of Human Leucocyte Interferon in non-Small Cell Lung Cancer." Abstract #715, *Proceedings*, Seventy-First Meeting of the American Association for Cancer Research/ Sixteenth Annual Meeting of the American Society of Clinical Oncology, 1980.

12. Moss, Ralph. *Cancer Syndrome*. New York: Grove Press, 1980.

13. Null, Gary, Robert Houston. "The Great Cancer Fraud." *Penthouse*: 11 (Sept. 1979), 76-82, 268-278.

14. Osserman, E. F., W. H. Sherman, R. Alexanian, J. T. Getterman, R. L. Humphrey. "Preliminary Results of the American Cancer Society Sponsored Trial of Human Leukocyte Interferon in Multiple Myeloma." Abstract #643, *Proceedings*. Seventy-First Annual Meeting of the American Association for Cancer Research/ Sixteenth Annual Meeting of the American Society of Clinical Oncology, 1980.

15. Rettig, Richard. *Cancer Crusade. The Story of the National Cancer Act of 1971*. Princeton: University of Princeton Press, 1977.

16. Rosenbaum, Ruth. "Cancer, Inc." *New Times*: 9 (11), 28-43, 1978.

17. Royhab, Ron. "Cancer Research Often Takes Back Seat." *Columbus* (Ohio) *Citizen Journal*: 19 (August 4, 1978), 1.

18. Saikowsky, Charlotte, Richard M. Harley. "Christian Healing: The Search for Answers." *Christian Science Monitor* (Mar. 14., 1979), 12-13.

19. Wade, Nicholas. "The Business of Science." *Science*: 207, 507, 1980.

APPENDIX

Hearing on United States Senate Bill 2043

On December 10, 1979 a hearing was held before the Subcommittee on Agricultural Research and General Legislation of the Committee on Agriculture, Nutrition, and Forestry. The subject was Bill No. 2043, "to provide for research in the diagnosis, prevention, and control of malignant tumors in domestic animals, poultry, and wildlife, with special emphasis on the role of CG."

We are reproducing this hearing because in it we hear some reputable scientists "testifying" to the scientific truth of what we have presented in this book. Further, it shows the conflict between the establishment scientists, confident that they have all the answers, and those who believe that the books are not yet closed, that basic innovative research, new ideas based upon solid demonstrable evidence, is still important in pushing back our obvious ignorance.

Since the main concern of our book has been cancer in humans, we have not indicated the importance of cancer in the world of birds, fishes, and mammals, domestic and wild. First of all, as the testimony indicates, loss of poultry and meat animals through cancer is considerable, with great loss to raisers of poultry and cattle. Second, cancer is one of the chief causes of death of domestic pets, and the possible health hazard of pet cancer has not been well investigated.

Senator John Melcher of Montana is a courageous, informed Senator with excellent scientific training and a degree in Veterinary Medicine. He has long been critical of the "war on cancer," and at least partly because of his reading of a version of this book, he introduced Senate Bill 2043 to provide money for the study of CG in cancers of poultry, domestic animals, and wildlife. Research of this kind can, of course, be of the first importance in the application to human cancers because of the CG synthesis by both animal and human cancer cells.

In a sense this hearing is a miniature drama, in which we see two opposing forces—the Department of Agriculture representatives, part of the established bureaucracy, on one side; and the outside scientists, although regarded as experts, on the other. The Hon. Donald W. Stewart from Alabama, chairman of the subcommittee, left after the opening statement in which this book manuscript was used as part of the introduction, and did not participate in the debate. The subcommittee felt that the qualifications of Senator Melcher being a veterinarian were sufficient to evaluate the matter for the entire subcommittee.

Representing the Department of Agriculture were Dr. T. B. Kinney, Jr., Associate Deputy Director of the Agricultural Research, Science and

Education Administration (SEA); John Victor, Chief, Budget Division; Dr. Graham Purchase, Acting Chief, livestock and veterinary science staff; Dr. Earl Splitter, principal veterinarian, Cooperative Research; and Dr. Douglas Bolt, animal physiologist, Agricultural Research.

Dr. Kinney's testimony made the following points:

1. Cancer is a major problem in domestic animals and poultry.
2. Progress has been made against Marek's disease (a kind of leukemia in poultry) and in cancer in mink.
3. The SEA has been studying CG—in reproduction!
4. The budget for CG-research is about six million. No additional money is necessary.

Artful questioning of Dr. Bolt by Senator Melcher brought out that most of the research done by the Department on cancer is applied rather than basic. Most cancer research is being done on mycotoxins as carcinogens (mycotoxins are derived from fungi).

Supporting the bill were Dr. Dale K. Sorensen, American Veterinary Medical Association and the Association of American Veterinary Colleges; Dr. Hernan Acevedo, Allegheny General Hospital, Pittsburgh; Dr. Michael Naughton, University of Colorado Hospital; Dr. Myron Blume, Mount Zion Hospital, San Francisco; and Dr. Vernon Stevens, Ohio State University Hospital, Columbus.

Dr. Sorenson makes an eloquent statement for

the need for money for research in cancer as proposed by the bill. He outlines the cost of animal and poultry cancer to the nation—some 26 million dollars a year.

He also points out that cancer is one of the chief causes of death among the dogs and cats we treasure as pets! Further, he states that virtually no money has been available in the veterinary colleges for the study of cancer! The only money from the NCI has been for animal cancers "demonstrating a potential human health hazard or an animal model of a similar cancer in man." No federal agency, he points out, is supporting research on cancer in wild birds and animals, poultry, and wild life. He also emphasizes the possible benefits of animal research in understanding human cancer.

The testimony of Drs. Acevedo and Naughton cover the basic information contained in this book about CG and also the crisis in funding research under the present system.

Dr. Blume suggests that cancer work on animals other than mice may be very valuable.

Dr. Stevens describes his long work with CG in the study of reproduction and describes his difficulty in obtaining funding in the United States for his work.

The hearing emphasizes again that any attempt to disturb the comfortable status quo in research is met with opposition and skepticism.

ANIMAL CANCER RESEARCH ACT

HEARING

BEFORE THE

SUBCOMMITTEE ON AGRICULTURAL RESEARCH AND GENERAL LEGISLATION

OF THE

COMMITTEE ON AGRICULTURE, NUTRITION, AND FORESTRY

UNITED STATES SENATE

NINETY-SIXTH CONGRESS

FIRST SESSION

ON

S. 2043

TO PROVIDE FOR RESEARCH IN THE DIAGNOSIS, PREVENTION, AND CONTROL OF MALIGNANT TUMORS IN DOMESTIC ANIMALS, POULTRY, AND WILDLIFE

DECEMBER 10, 1979

Printed for the use of the
Committee on Agriculture, Nutrition, and Forestry

U.S. GOVERNMENT PRINTING OFFICE
57-174 O WASHINGTON : 1980

COMMITTEE ON AGRICULTURE, NUTRITION, AND FORESTRY

HERMAN E. TALMADGE, Georgia, *Chairman*

GEORGE McGOVERN, South Dakota
WALTER D. HUDDLESTON, Kentucky
RICHARD B. STONE, Florida
PATRICK J. LEAHY, Vermont
EDWARD ZORINSKY, Nebraska
JOHN MELCHER, Montana
DONALD W. STEWART, Alabama
DAVID H. PRYOR, Arkansas

DAVID L. BOREN, Oklahoma
JESSIE HELMS, North Carolina
MILTON R. YOUNG, North Dakota
BOB DOLE, Kansas
S. I. HAYAKAWA, California
RICHARD G. LUGAR, Indiana
THAD COCHRAN, Mississippi
RUDY BOSCHWITZ, Minnesota
ROGER W. JEPSEN, Iowa

Henry J. Casso, *Staff Director*
Carl P. Rose, *General Counsel*
George S. Dunlop, *Minority Staff Director*

SUBCOMMITTEE ON AGRICULTURE RESEARCH AND GENERAL LEGISLATION

DONALD W. STEWART, Alabama, *Chairman*

PATRICK J. LEAHY, Vermont
RICHARD B. STONE, Florida
HERMAN E. TALMADGE, Georgia
RICHARD G. LUGAR, Indiana

BOB DOLE, Kansas
MILTON R. YOUNG, North Dakota
RUDY BOSCHWITZ, Minnesota

Contents

CHRONOLOGICAL LIST OF WITNESSES

APPENDIX

ANIMAL CANCER RESEARCH ACT

(S. 2043)

Monday, December 10, 1979

U.S. SENATE,
SUBCOMMITTEE ON AGRICULTURAL RESEARCH
AND GENERAL LEGISLATION OF THE
COMMITTEE ON AGRICULTURE, NUTRITION,
AND FORESTRY,
Washington, D.C.

The subcommittee met, pursuant to notice, at 9:55 a.m., in room 324, Russell Senate Office Building, Hon. Donald W. Stewart (chairman of the subcommittee) presiding.

Present: Senator Stewart.

Also present: Senator Melcher.

STATEMENT OF HON. DONALD W. STEWART, A U.S. SENATOR FROM ALABAMA

Senator STEWART. We will call the meeting to order.

This subcommittee convenes this morning to hear testimony on S. 2043,[1] introduced by Senator Melcher, a bill to provide for research in the diagnosis, prevention, and control of malignant tumors in domestic animals, poultry, and wildlife.

The scientists and veterinarians at the Department of Agriculture have made a number of vital contributions recently in preventing and controlling animal disease.

At one time, avian leukosis, also known as Marek's disease, cost the poultry industry over $200 million each year. With the discovery of a vaccine to treat this type of cancer, loss to the poultry industry has been reduced to $30 million per year. USDA has made great strides in the detection of bovine leukemia, a strain of cancer similar to that which can afflict man, and which costs the cattle industry $20 million per year. Research continues on this disease, but in the meantime, the Department of Agriculture has discovered a useful diagnostic test which aids in the identification of carriers of the disease. Other areas which the Science and Education Administration at USDA is currently researching include cancer eye, a malignancy affecting beef cattle mainly in the Midwest; pulmonary adenomatosis, a lung cancer which afflicts sheep; and mycotoxins, a known human carcinogen which can be toxic to animals and which, at the least, can depress animal immune mechanisms making that animal more susceptible to other diseases.

---

[1] See pages 240 and 241 for the text of S. 2043 and staff explanation of S. 2043.

As a veterinarian and a U.S. Senator, my colleague, Senator Melcher is doubly qualified to introduce such a bill as this. He has a long history of interest in the progress of cancer research in this country not only in farm animals, but in humans as well. I laud the Senator for his abiding interest and efforts in this area.

Due to a prior commitment, I will be unable to remain for the hearing today, and turn the Chair over to my able colleague from Montana. I would like to assure you, Senator Melcher, that this subcommittee will give full consideration to the views expressed here today as it considers the piece of legislation before it.

Thank you, Senator Melcher.

STATEMENT OF HON. JOHN MELCHER, A U.S. SENATOR FROM MONTANA

Senator MELCHER [presiding]. Thank you very much, Senator.

In the United States, after billions of dollars have been spent on research through the National Cancer Institute to alleviate cancer, only relatively limited results have been attained. Human cancer research has received more public funding than any other medical research being conducted by the National Institutes of Health. Yet the results from basic research in terms of prevention or cure have been very limited.

As a contrast, the research on cancer involving animals and poultry conducted by the Department of Agriculture through its Science and Education Administration with comparatively miniscule funding has yielded some positive results in the control in poultry of neurolymphomatosis gallinarum, commonly known as Marek's disease. A successful vaccine has been developed that prevents this type of cancer in poultry.

While it should be emphasized at the outset that the scientists working within the Department of Agriculture and the National Cancer Institute cooperate to the fullest extent, it is apparent that a funding disparity exists between the two, comparable to David and Goliath.

The Department of Agriculture's Science and Education Administration will testify that approximately $6 million is being spent annually on cancer-related problems in domestic animals. In the budget process developed by the executive branch over the past several years the Department of Agriculture has not been pressing for rapid or gigantic increases in appropriations for this purpose. However, a comparison of the amounts appropriated for the basic research on cancer between the Science and Education Administration and the National Cancer Institute leads me to state emphatically that an increase in basic research work on cancer in animals should definitely be granted.

Finding the keys to unlock the puzzle of what causes cancer or how it can be prevented is related in animals and man. Successful research on man, animals, or birds will begin to unravel the unknown on cancer for all of them.

There have been complaints for several years that the National Cancer Institute has not adequately considered some basic cancer research areas. Dr. Bob Netterberg—not a researcher himself but a dentist by profession—has consistently argued over the past several years that recognition of some previous research, chorionic gonadotrophin has been ignored by the National Cancer Institute; that very little attention has been paid by the National Cancer Institute to grant applications by researchers in this and other areas. Dr. Netterberg has documented these facts in his recent publication, "The Road Not Taken: Toward a Cancer Vaccine."[1]

S. 2043 was introduced a few weeks ago to provide more emphasis through the Science and Education Administration for basic research on cancer in animals. Specifically, the bill directs emphasis on basic research on common agents found in many types of cancer such as chorionic gonadotrophin. While the Science and Education Administration has an ongoing program of researching the physiology of chorionic gonadotrophin, it has not attempted the research on the basis of its linkage as an agent with animal cancers. The bill specifically is intended to develop basic research on cancer in this area. It is a small start—a very late start—but a start that is needed immediately.

Our first witness this morning will be Dr. T. B. Kinney, Jr., Associate Deputy Director, Agricultural Research, Science and Education Administration, of the U.S. Department of Agriculture.

---

1. See p. 242.

STATEMENT OF DR. T. B. KINNEY, JR., ASSOCIATE DEPUTY DIRECTOR, AGRICULTURAL RESEARCH, SCIENCE, AND EDUCATION ADMINISTRATION, U.S. DEPARTMENT OF AGRICULTURE, ACCOMPANIED BY JOHN VICTOR, CHIEF BUDGET DIVISION; DR. GRAHAM PURCHASE, ACTING CHIEF, LIVESTOCK AND VETERINARY SCIENCE STAFF; DR. EARL V. SPLITTER, PRINCIPAL VETERINARIAN, COOPERATIVE RESEARCH; AND DR. DOUGLAS BOLT, ANIMAL PHYSIOLOGIST, AGRICULTURAL RESEARCH

Dr. KINNEY. Mr. Chairman and members of the subcommittee, thank you for the opportunity to testify on S. 2043, the Animal Cancer Research Act, and the research on malignant tumors which the Science and Education Administration (SEA) is conducting.

I am accompanied by Mr. John Victor, Chief, Budget Division, SEA; Dr. Graham Purchase, DVM, Ph. D., Acting Chief, Livestock and Veterinarian Science Staff, Science and Education Administration/Agricultural Research (SEA/AR); Dr. Earl J. Splitter, DVM, principal veterinarian, Science and Education Administration, Cooperative Research (SEA/CR); and Dr. Douglas Bolt, animal physiologist, SEA/AR.

The Department supports the intent of this legislation. However, the Department has adequate authorization and funding for this research, and does not believe that enactment of S. 2043 is necessary. The Department does recognize that some aspects of cancer research could possibly be more intensively reviewed. However, we are not prepared to ask for additional authorization at this time.

Losses in livestock and poultry caused by malignancies have been of continuing concern to the Department. In 1978, tumorous conditions resulted in the loss of millions of pounds of federally inspected meat animals and poultry because of condemnations at time of slaughter. This does not include the very substantial but unmeasured losses due to reduced productivity and deaths occurring from malignancies in animals on the farm.

Intensive research efforts by the Science and Education Administration (SEA) and its cooperators in the past decade have led to major breakthroughs in controlling several of the most important causes of malignancies in farm animals, Cancer viruses and cancer cells have been grown artificially in culture and their chemical and antigenic makeup determined. Mechanisms of virus and cell replication have been studied and compared with replication in other viruses and normal cells.

From these discoveries the mechanism of transmission has been better understood and diagnostic tests have been developed. Marek's disease of poultry—a leukemia-like malignancy—has been found to be caused by a virus.

This discovery led to the development of a vaccine which has resulted in annual losses from the disease formerly at $200 million being reduced now to about $30 million.

The mechanism of the protection has been

shown to be mediated by both cellular and humoral responses against new antigens that are characteristic of and appear in tumor cells.

Leukemia in cattle also has been found to be of viral origin and technology has been developed which will lead to reduction and perhaps eventual elimination of the disease. SEA research also has determined the cause and provided means for controlling the malignancy-like disease of mink known as Aleutian disease. This was a major cause of loss in the production of mink for fur.

Despite these advances, other formidable malignancy problems of livestock and poultry remain to be solved. SEA currently—fiscal year 1980—is allocating $6 million for this research.

The Science and Education Administration in cooperation with other Federal agencies and other institutions has a significant program in basic research on cancer in animals. This includes studies on the genetics of the immune response, possible etiologic agents of different kinds of cancer, the effects of these agents on the host genetic materials that change in the process of becoming cancerous, mechanisms by which the control of cell proliferation of cancerous cells is lost, and new antigens, receptors, and other substances on the surface of cancer cells.

Other efforts by SEA and its cooperators to solve animal malignancies include studies to prevent cancer-eye in cattle and pulmonary adenomatosis in sheep. More effective methods are being sought to reduce or eliminate leukemia of cattle and Marek's disease and lymphoid leukosis of poultry. In addition, studies are in progress on mechanisms occurring in animals that affect natural and acquired immunity to malignancies. Promising substances are being evaluated that show suppressant action against the multiplication of animal tumor cells.

Another major effort is centering on the problem of mycotoxins, a group of known carcinogens for man and possible carcinogens and known toxicants for farm animals. Methods are being sought to eliminate these carcinogens from food and feeds. A portion of the basic research program on mycotoxins is related to cancer in animals including the effect of mycotoxins on the cellular and humoral immune response, the ability of animals to resist disease, the ability of animals to respond to vaccines and the effect of mycotoxins on cellular genetic components that results in cancer.

SEA has a strong program on cancer in animals and basic research on animal reproduction. These programs give high priority to solving problems of significant economic importance in farm animals. We are not proposing to reduce any of these high priority programs.

SEA has ongoing programs on the endocrinology of reproduction involving pituitary and gonadal hormones. Chorionic gonadotrophin causes ovulation as does the pituitary luteinizing hormone which is important in farm animals. Chorionic gonadotrophin is used extensively in research as a tool, often in combination with other hormones, to regulate ovarian function.

Some of the possible research approaches are the clarification of the nature of the hormone chorionic gonadotrophin and the mechanisms of its action including its role in stimulation of cell proliferation and its possible role in the acceptance or rejection by the animal of embryo cells or cancer cells.

We agree with statements in S. 2043 that basic research on malignant tumors is essential to the health of animals; that such research may be beneficial in determining whether there are common factors which may cause malignancies in both man and animals, and that all carcinogenic agents have not been adequately identified in domestic animals.

We believe there have been and continue to be well-coordinated efforts to solve the malignancies of food animals which cause major economic losses. The health-related research programs of SEA are regularly reviewed and adjusted as necessary to assure that attention is being directed to the most important problems. The successes just referred to in this testimony in controlling Marek's disease in poultry and in solving the cause of leukemia in cattle did not result from isolated studies, but were due to well-coordinated efforts by SEA and its cooperators.

These efforts resulted in advances of substantial significance to veterinary as well as medical science. This included the first cancerous disease for which a successful, commercially applicable vaccine was ever developed and the vaccine is now applied worldwide. Another major advance included conclusive proof of the viral cause of leukemia in cattle—a question not completely resolved as yet in the similar disease of human leukemia.

In conclusion, we believe that current authorizations are adequate for continued, productive studies by SEA on malignancies of food animals; $6 million of the $74.4 million of SEA's fiscal 1980 appropriation for animal protection research, or more than 8 percent of that money, is currently being spent on malignancy research.

We would expect to be spending at least the same amount in fiscal year 1981. Given the basic nature of the research involved, research is being conducted in other Federal agencies directed toward these same underlying factors.

Mr. Chairman, thank you very much for the opportunity to testify before your subcommittee. My colleagues and I will be glad to answer your questions.

Senator MELCHER. Dr. Bolt, so far as the intensive research efforts by the Science and Education Administration, it has been connected with the problem of domestic animals or poultry, and in looking at that problem, and in trying to alleviate the losses on an economic basis, is that correct? Is that an accurate statement?

Dr. BOLT. Yes.

Senator MELCHER. So when you get the economic loss, you look at that problem and say: "Let's find a way to resolve it or to alleviate it or to minimize it." Then you go to basic research at that point; is that correct?

Dr. BOLT. That approach is used. However it is sometimes more efficient to first see if the applied approach might solve the problem. Then if that is not successful, go to basic research.

Senator MELCHER. For instance, in the complete

leukosis problem in poultry, it is a combination, is it not, the vaccine for Marek's disease is part of it, and hygenic prevention is also a part of it?

Dr. BOLT. That is correct.

Dr. PURCHASE. That is correct.

Senator MELCHER. So you come from the start, here is a problem that costs money. Let's see how we can alleviate it, minimize it.

When basic research gets into it, well and good. But if you could alleviate it without the basic research, that is about where you would stop?

Dr. BOLT. If the applied approach will solve the problem, yes.

Senator MELCHER. While the testimony dwells on the problems connected with food animals, you did mention the mink and what you call the Aleutian disease. You got into that because of an economic problem of people who produced mink for fur, which is not a food of course.

That is also a part of it, is it not?

Dr. KINNEY. Yes. I think research on fur-bearing animals comes under the purview of the Department of Agriculture insofar as fur bearing animals are raised domestically for income purposes.

Senator MELCHER. There is one obvious handicap. As far as basic research is concerned, you do not start with the basic research when you get into it. What was the term you used, applied?

Dr. BOLT. Applied approach, yes.

Senator MELCHER. While I am sure that the Science and Education Administration has been diligent on this, the bill would attempt to have you go a little bit beyond that into basic research itself.

Do you find any problem with that, if you went beyond this applied approach? There is an economic cost, let's see how we can alleviate it. Do you find any problem in the Department with, "Let's do a little broader basic research"?

Dr. BOLT. We are involved with both basic and applied research. For the most part, we use the applied approach first, and if it is not satisfactory, we proceed to a more basic approach.

Senator MELCHER. Well, the bill attempts to change that a little bit. The bill dwells on the fact that basic research is essential, that some types of basic research have not been adequately pursued, gets into coordination, and states "that significant theories of a common factor in malignant tumors, such as chorionic gonadotrophin, have not been pursued in depth."

So the bill really does not start by saying, we have a huge economic loss in certain areas. The bill starts on the premise that we are not doing enough basic research. That is a little bit of a different start for the Science and Education Administration than what you have been doing before, because you have identified the economic loss and said, perhaps we can alleviate that by various applied means, not basic research.

Dr. BOLT. Yes, it is different. We try not to spend effort to solve a problem that does not exist.

But there are certainly many problems in the area that I am familiar with, which is reproduction, that need a basic research approach.

Dr. KINNEY. If I might interject, I think in most of our research, and particularly our research on reproduction, somewhere between 40 and 50 percent of the funds are devoted to basic research. In this case, I think approximately $2.4 million of the $6 million is actually what we would classify as basic research.

Senator MELCHER. The bill, first of all, identifies basic research as not being sufficient in terms of animal cancer and research, and second, authorizes funds to augment it.

One other point: You have not been given any direction in terms of wildlife. I will use that term in its broadest sense, which would include wild birds. And while the mink research you have done would relate itself to both domestic mink—I do not know if we even call them domestic.

Dr. KINNEY. I may have used that term a little broadly. I meant to refer to fur-bearing animals.

Senator MELCHER. Yes, that are in captivity and that are ranched; I think that is the best term, for income. You have not been given any direction to look at wildlife, and again, I use that term in its broadest sense, including wild birds.

Is that a problem?

Dr. KINNEY. I would ask one of my colleagues to respond. But I might say that we are not precluded from looking at wildlife insofar as it relates to vectors or reservoirs of domestic diseases or because they simply may be a good research animal.

Dr. Purchase, would you comment further and perhaps with respect to the fact that we do research on any animals, including those related to exotic disease transmission.

Dr. PURCHASE. That is correct; where the wildlife or vectors play an important role in domestic diseases, we are heavily involved. In our turkey-raising areas, we have found influenza infections are introduced by wild ducks, migrating ducks. And we are doing considerable work on the role of wild ducks in causing the influenza outbreaks in turkeys.

That is one of many examples.

Senator MELCHER. I am well aware that we are going to carefully husband and probably limit any basic research in wildlife. But, again, I come to the point of the basic research, not necessarily being related to anything economic, but it is the basic research for the purpose of the search for knowledge, the most basic type of research, which is not motivated necessarily at all by economic considerations, but which is only motivated by search of knowledge.

I think that that is perhaps a much broader direction than what the Science and Education Administration has had before in the Department of Agriculture. It is one that I believe we need a modest increase in, entirely in that direction.

So the bill attempts to emphasize that approach, rather than simply looking at the economics of it. In doing so, as first-named author of this bill, and the introducer of the bill, on the basis of the feeling that we are not using all our capability in basic cancer research; we are attempting to allow and to direct another branch of the Federal Government with competence to enter into cancer research on the basic level, rather than just on the basis of the economic returns involved with animals or poultry.

In regard to your grant program, about half of your $6 million is spent on the basis of the grants to other institutions, other than within the Department of Agriculture?

Mr. VICTOR. Of the total of $6 million, $3.3 million is in-house in the USDA laboratories.

Senator MELCHER. Within, which would be where?

Mr. VICTOR. There is $1.3 million in research on avian leukosis underway in Pullman, Wash., and East Lansing, Mich.

Senator MELCHER. Wait a minute; this is not in-house?

Mr. VICTOR. This is in SEA's research laboratories. There is almost a half-million dollars of research on bovine leukemia in Ames, Iowa, and Pullman, Wash. There is also better than a million and a half of work currently underway in the area of mycotoxins.

Senator MELCHER. That is in-house?

Mr. VICTOR. That is in-house. In addition, there is considerable work in the various State agricultural experimental stations.

Senator MELCHER. That would be at the land-grant colleges?

Mr. VICTOR. The major portion of the extramural program is at the land-grant colleges. A minor portion is in the area of special research grants.

So the bulk of the work is either in the SEA-owned and operated research laboratories, and/or the State experimental stations.

Senator MELCHER. What type of criteria do you have for any grants to any of the other research centers that are not within the Department of Agriculture?

Dr. SPLITTER. We have several programs that would allow research or provide for research in extramural institutions. We have a special program in animal health that provides funding for veterinary colleges as well as experiment stations.

Some of this money is being used in a special competitive grant program, which includes mycotoxin research projects, placed by competition. Some of the formula grant programs in animal health are being used for cancer research at experiment stations such as Nevada, Utah, and Texas.

So these are some of the examples of how funds are placed outside the Department by formula and by competitive means.

Senator MELCHER. When you say competitive means, how do you handle that?

Dr. SPLITTER. In the last several years, we have had specific amounts of money appropriated for animal health research. We have advisory committees that indicate the priorities in animal health research.

These priorities then are identified as eligible areas for competition by veterinary college personnel, or experiment stations, or any university scientists who have competence in the eligible areas of research.

The availability of money is advertised in the Federal Register. Proposals are received, and then peer panels of experts in these various subject areas evaluate proposals and recommend those proposals to the Department which they feel will accomplish the most for the money; these are then funded on that basis for periods of from 1 to 5 years.

Senator MELCHER. About how much—could you give me a figure of how much is going into the grants?

Dr. SPLITTER. The total extramural program includes about $2.7 million, of which the special research grants portion is $127,000.

Senator MELCHER. Of the $6 million?

Dr. SPLITTER. Yes.

Senator MELCHER. And that is mostly for work on mycotoxins?

Dr. SPLITTER. About $2.3 million of the total extramural program is for mycotoxin research, including the $127,000 special research grants.

Senator MELCHER. And then also cancer eye?

Dr. SPLITTER. The total extramural program is $34,000 in cancer eye research.

Senator MELCHER. Is there another area besides the mycotoxins and cancer eye? Is that it on the grants?

Dr. SPLITTER. The extramural program includes $268,000 on avian leukosis and there is research on bovine leukemia which is considerably less. None of this is special research grants.

Senator MELCHER. Those four areas then?

Dr. SPLITTER. Yes.

Senator MELCHER. Now, Dr. Bolt, on the physiology of chorionic gonadotrophin, where is that work being done?

Dr. BOLT. Let me clarify. I don't know of research in the Department where chorionic gonadotrophin is the central focus of a research problem. Chorionic gonadotrophin is used widely by many researchers, particularly in reproduction, as a research tool, because of its biologic properties.

For the most part, it is used because it has important biologic properties that mimic those of pituitary hormones. The pituitary hormone is much less available.

Chorionic gonadotrophin (HCG) can be extracted from the urine of pregnant women. The basic research on chorionic gonadotrophin has been conducted, not because we are studying exactly what does chorionic gonadotrophin do, but we are studying the basic actions of the hormone; the goal being to understand the mechanisms responsible for the stimulation and production of progesterone, the hormone necessary to maintain pregnancy.

HCG is used where one needs to mimic the biologic action of luteinizing hormones. It is quite commonly used experimentally to ovulate sows at a precise time. Such a procedure certainly may have an economic advantage.

HCG is used to cause ovulation in cattle, and to aid in estrogen synchronization programs, or efforts to increase the number of ovulations animals might have.

Senator MELCHER. Referring to this sentence on the bottom of page 2, second from the bottom paragraph:

> Some of the research problems are in the clarification of the nature of the hormone, chorionic gonadotrophin, and the mechanisms of its action, including

its role in the stimulation of cell proliferation and its possible role in the acceptance or rejection by the animal of embryo cells or cancer cells.

Dr. BOLT. I cannot speak for the entire Department as to what is going on, but I can speak to some of that, particularly the mechanisms of action, and the role of stimulating cells to proliferate.

One of the actions of chorionic gonadotrophin, as well as luteinizing hormone, is to transfer a follicle into a corpus luteum, a process called luteinization.

I really can't address that last part of the question because I have not studied cancer. Absence of rejection of embryo cells implies the maintenance of pregnancy or the maintenance of a condition that is necessary for pregnancy, which chorionic gonadotrophin certainly has this function in humans, and a similar action can be demonstrated as in normal animals.

This has been studied in an effort to reveal the mechanisms responsible for maintenance of pregnancies. We try to answer questions such as, how does the female actually know she is pregnant? This mechanism is not really known.

Dr. PURCHASE. The paragraph was intended to show some of the problems that could be approached using our technology, our research, and our expertise.

Senator MELCHER. In other words, that is intended to show that——

Dr. PURCHASE. These are some of the research problems.

Senator MELCHER. Which you could go beyond, into which you are not now in.

Dr. PURCHASE. That is correct.

Senator MELCHER. That is one of the attempts of the bill, basically to authorize additional funds so that is possible.

I do recognize that none of the work you are now doing you want to see decreased; in other words, taking some of the $6 million and taking it away from what you are now doing to pursue something that might be required if this bill is passed.

Thank you all very much. I appreciate your testimony.

The next witness will be Dr. Dale K. Sorensen, representing the American Veterinary Medical Association, and the Association of American Veterinary Medical Colleges.

STATEMENT OF DALE K. SORENSEN, D.V.M. AND PH. D., REPRESENTING THE AMERICAN VETERINARY MEDICAL ASSOCIATION AND THE ASSOCIATION OF AMERICAN VETERINARY MEDICAL COLLEGES

Dr. SORENSEN. Mr. Chairman and members of the subcommittee, the American Veterinary Medical Association and the Association of American Veterinary Medical Colleges appreciate this opportunity to appear before the subcommittee in support of S. 2043.

I am a member of the American Veterinary Medical Association's Council on Research, and I am chairman of the Department of Large Animal

Clinical Sciences, College of Veterinary Medicine, at the University of Minnesota.

I speak for the American Veterinary Medical Association, which represents about 32,000 member veterinarians and the Association of American Veterinary Medical Colleges, which represents the 23 colleges of veterinary medicine and the departments of veterinary science of the colleges of agriculture in the United States.

It is a pleasure for me to present a brief summary of cancer in animals, and the impact that this problem has in the United States.

Cancer is a disease not unique to man. It knows no species barriers, affecting all species of domestic animals, wildlife, and poultry.

Various types of tumors have been encountered in many vertebrate species, including mammals, birds, and reptiles. Fish are also susceptible to this disease.

There is a greater concern of cancer in the domestic species of animals than in the nondomesticated since it has a greater impact on man and our quality of life. Cancer in animals and poultry affects the food supply of the Nation, as affected animals or birds cannot be utilized for human consumption.

Malignant tumors in companion animals or pets cause disruption to family life as well as cost consumers considerable expense for veterinary medical care to manage the ill patient. The potential public health hazard of animal neoplasia is of concern and needs greater definition.

There is an urgent need to increase the emphasis of cancer research on domestic animals and poultry. The primary basis for this need is to develop better methods for the diagnosis, control, and prevention of cancer in food producing animals and poultry.

There is also a need for improved diagnostic and therapeutic methods for cancer of companion animals. Companion animals play an extremely important role in maintaining the mental health of millions of Americans. Pets are essential members of families and necessary for happiness and a high quality of life for many people. It is also well recognized that animals provide excellent models for biomedical research in oncology. Increased knowledge of animal oncology will lead to a greater utilization of animals in solving human cancer problems.

A better understanding of the needs for additional funds to conduct research on neoplasia may be gained by reviewing some data.

Prevalence of neoplasms in food animals and poultry: Reliable data are available on the prevalence of neoplasms in food producing animals and poultry from the Federal meat and poultry inspection program, Food Safety and Quality Service, U.S. Department of Agriculture. Animals and birds sent to slaughter are subjected to ante mortem and post mortem inspection to ensure wholesomeness for human consumption. The following tables provide data on the prevalence of animal neoplasms for 1978.

I will not go through the tables, but just note that in cattle we have the most neoplasms, and the three big disease problems are carcinoma, epithelioma, leukosis and sarcoma.

TABLE 1.—NUMBER OF ANIMAL CARCASSES CONDEMNED FOR NEOPLASIA IN 1978

Neoplasm	Species				
	Cattle	Calves	Sheep	Swine	Horses
Carcinoma	3,303	7	31	444	36
Epithelioma	16,833	38	3	104	3
Leukosis (leukemia)	7,945	128	42	1,316	15
Sarcoma	325	10	8	835	119
Miscellaneous	316	16	7	632	41
Total	29,222	199	91	3,331	214

We also have to keep in mind that any carcass which has neoplasia is condemned, not fit for human consumption. And on table 2 we have listed the number of animal carcasses with parts removed due to neoplasia, where only parts of animal carcasses are not utilized for human consumption.

TABLE 2.—NUMBER OF ANIMAL CARCASSES WITH PARTS REMOVED DUE TO NEOPLASIA

Neoplasm	Species				
	Cattle	Calves	Sheep	Swine	Horses
Epithelioma	75,267	328	190	295	3
Miscellaneous	2,059	23	5	994	64
Total	77,326	351	195	1,289	67

The biggest neoplasm is epithelioma. We have also listed on table 3 the number of birds and percent condemned for neoplasia for calendar year 1978.

As one can note from the table, the largest category is young chickens, where approximately 1 percent of the total birds slaughtered in calender year 1978 were condemned for this particular disease.

TABLE 3.—NUMBER OF BIRDS AND PERCENT CONDEMNED FOR NEOPLASIA DURING CALENDAR YEAR 1978

Class of poultry	Leukosis	
	Number	Percent of total
Young chickens	3,633,324	0.10
Mature chickens	308,375	.16
Fryer/roaster turkeys	253	(1)
Young turkeys	2,425	(1)
Old turkeys	112	.01
Ducks	286	(1)
Other poultry	11	(1)
Total	3,944,786	

[1] Less than one-hundreth of 1 percent—Fourth leading cause of poultry condemnations.

The data presented in these three tables provide some useful information on the importance of neoplastic diseases in food producing animals and poultry in the United States. It should also be kept in mind that this represents only the animals and birds that were processed through federally inspected plants in the United States. The percent of animals and birds slaughtered in federally inspected plants varies with each animal species and ranges from approximately 86 to 96 percent.

I would like to comment that we have many thousands of birds and animals which die from various melanomas that are not sent to federally inspected plants. Many go to rendering plants or are disposed of in other fashion.

For example, we recently conducted a study on leukosis cases in Minnesota and what percent went to inspected plants and what percent were disposed of using other channels. Approximately 50 percent of these animals were disposed of other than through meat processing plants.

So it is difficult to say other than this represents some fairly conservative estimate of the total numbers of these tumors that occur each year.

The economic loss due to cancer in food animals and poultry can be estimated utilizing meat and poultry inspection service data on the number of animal carcasses or parts of carcasses condemned for neoplasms. It is also necessary to include the economic loss associated with veterinary medical services for a portion of these animals.

For example, many livestock producers will have utilized veterinary medical services to diagnose the animal's disease problem. In the case of squamous cell carcinoma of the eye, the most prevalent neoplastic disease of cattle, surgical treatment is frequently employed. There is also an indirect loss associated with premature or unscheduled loss of animals from the breeding herd as it may reduce potential productivity of the herd.

I should add that there are losses of economic activity, prior to the time the animal is lost from the herd, through loss of milk production or failure to gain weight—so if we look at these 3 years, and estimate the economic loss, I have come up with a conservative estimate. It is approximately $17,500,000 of loss due to contamination of animal carcasses or parts; $4,500,000 in loss due to condemnation of poultry; $2 million of loss associated with decreased productivity; and $2 million of loss associated with veterinary medical care, for a total of $26 million.

This figure represents a conservative assessment of the annual economic loss associated with cancer of food producing animals and poultry. It is recognized that the carcasses condemned are utilized for other nonhuman products, but all carcasses condemned represent a direct total loss to the producer and, ultimately, to the consumer in higher prices for the product.

In food producing animals and poultry there are three economically important neoplastic diseases. In cattle, the two important diseases are bovine leukosis—leukemia—and squamous cell carcinoma of the eye. The prevalence of squamous cell carcinoma in adult Hereford cattle may be as high as 20 to 30 percent, and it represents the leading cause of condemnations at slaughter. In the case of bovine leukosis—leukemia—serologic studies suggest that approximately 20 percent of adult dairy cattle are infected with the leukemia virus necessary for the disease to develop. Meat inspection data show that this is the second leading neoplastic disease.

Another cause of economic loss is associated with the export of purebred cattle. In 1978, the United States exported 122,000 breeding cattle with a value of $94 million. Some potential importing countries, for example Yugoslavia, prohibit the import of U.S. cattle due to the presence of bovine leukemia virus infection in dairy herds. In the future, we may be unable to export breeding cattle to foreign countries with control programs for leukosis unless we have a similar level of control.

Both of these diseases are very prevalent diseases by any standard used for comparison.

In the case of poultry, the most common neoplastic disease is Marek's disease. Prior to the development and use of a vaccine, Marek's disease constituted an extremely serious economic threat to the poultry industry. Losses were estimated to be in excess of $150 million annually in the United States. Losses still occur because the vaccines are not 100 percent effective, and there is concern about the emergence of more pathogenic strains of the virus.

Neoplasms in companion animals: Companion animals such as dogs and cats frequently develop cancer. In fact, the prevalence is greater in companion animals than in food producing animals because the life span of farm animals is shorter than for pets, and there is less time for diseases of old age, such as neoplasms, to be expressed.

The occurrence of cancer in dogs and cats is similar to that in man with some species differences. The prevalence of tumors in dogs and cats has been subjected to several studies. The occurrence of tumors in dogs and cats hospitalized in veterinary teaching hospitals in 12 veterinary colleges in the United States was reported for a 5-year period—1964 to 1969. This study revealed a 5.5 percent incidence of tumors in over 100,000 hospitalized canine patients. Malignancy is one of the most important causes of death in dogs.

There is an urgent need for research to develop improved methods in cancer diagnosis and therapy. Veterinary oncology is just developing and needs research findings to improve the quality of care for patients and for the control of these diseases. One cannot assess an economic value on the problem of cancer in companion animals or the cost of providing veterinary medical care for these animals, but it certainly involves several millions of dollars annually.

I would like to add that it is difficult to get research funds to do any research on the whole issue of cancer in companion animals unless one can demonstrate a human health relatedness to it. So this restricts and limits the amount of funds which is available for research in this particular area.

Cancer in zoo animals, wildlife and fish: Neoplasia have been reported in virtually all animal phyla. The incidence rates of tumors encountered in this broad range of species has not been studied. There is little information available except for reports of various tumors in the many species of mammals, birds, reptiles, and fish. Funds are needed for research to provide more information on the extent of neoplasms in this group and to develop approaches for cancer therapy in zoo animals.

Human health hazards of animal cancer: There is no evidence as yet that the bovine leukemia virus poses any danger to man. This virus infects sheep and goats, and it is oncogenic in sheep. Investigators have not found antibodies to bovine leukemia virus in the sera of cancer patients or of normal humans from high risk groups. At the present, bovine leukemia virus is an adulterant in our meat and milk which could be prevented if additional technology were known. The virus can be propagated in mammalian cells and nonhuman primates. This has caused concern in the scientific community. There has been similar concern with Marek's disease. There is no evidence linking this disease with human infection or cancer, but further studies are probably warranted.

Role of animal cancer for biomedical research: Animals with spontaneous neoplasms can and do play an important role in the total cancer research program. They serve as models for investigations that cannot be carried out in man. Increased knowledge and understanding of cancer in animals will increase the use of animals as models for the study of cancer in man.

In summary, we believe that there is a need for providing funds for research on cancer problems in domestic animals, poultry, and wildlife. We believe that an urgent need exists from both economic and humanitarian viewpoints. We believe that it will be a good investment and that future cost-benefit analysis will be able to demonstrate it in the area of food producing animals and poultry.

Certainly, the cost-benefit ratio of Marek's disease is an excellent example of the potential that may exist.

We have some concern that the level of funding proposed in the bill is not adequate to really provide for the level of thrust intended in the Animal Cancer Research Act. We are in total support of this bill to provide for research in the diagnosis, prevention, and control of malignant tumors in domestic animals, poultry, and wildlife.

There is a great concern among veterinary colleges and veterinary research departments of the lack of research funds to conduct research on cancer problems in animals. Currently, in general, there are only two major potential Federal sources of support to fund such research. The National Cancer Institute provides support for projects on animal cancer demonstrating either a potential human health hazard or an animal model of a similar type of cancer in man. This severely limits the type of ongenic research which is eligible for NCI funding. The other source is the Science and Education Administration (SEA), of the U.S. Department of Agriculture. They have supported research on economically important neoplastic diseases of animals and poultry in the past and indicate continued support for economically important cancer programs. Funding levels for animal health research and disease priorities restrict and limit the cancer disease problems that are eligible for funding from SEA. In assessing the situation there is no Federal granting agency that is supporting research on cancer in animals or birds with emphasis on protecting the health of domestic animals, poultry, and wildlife. It is believed that basic research on animal cancer will also lead to a better understanding of all types of cancer. The potential benefit of this type of research to assist in solving the human cancer problem would be greatly increased.

We thank you for the opportunity to express our views.

Senator MELCHER. Dr. Sorensen, you touched on a significant point, I believe, the motivation for this bill, when you were talking about companion animals, that you cannot assess an economic value on the problem of cancer in companion animals.

What is their life worth? For the person who has companion animals, there is no way of assessing economic value to that life, and you add it is difficult to receive funds for this because you cannot link it to an economic cost, and cannot link it to whether it is a hazard to human health.

I think that is a good point. We do not know if cancer in these companion animals can somehow be linked to human health. We ought to find out, because they are with us, in setting aside the sentimental feelings for the animals, setting, that aside, the other aspect of whether or not it is related to human health is extremely important, because we are exposed to them every day.

That is what we would like to do in this bill, start looking not just at economic matters, look first of all at basic research to see—what we can find out for the sake of knowledge, and if what we find out in basic research can lead us to a prevention and cure of any of these various types of cancer, we would be that much enhanced.

A lot of our great breakthroughs have occurred through our knowledge of animals. Jenner, didn't he develop the smallpox vaccine after he found out that milkmaids in England had a protection against it, and then linked that unknown protection against smallpox from the fact that they were milking cows that often had cowpox and developed an immunity. Is that the way?

Dr. SORENSEN. Yes; that is an excellent example of the role animal cancer has played. It was the first viral vaccine. It was the result of an observation made in animal cancer.

I sincerely believe that there is just a wealth of resource material out there if we would start looking at the animal cancers and investigate them just for the basic knowledge and information that can be generated, that can be applicable to human neoplasias.

There are many of these animal cancers that do not appear to be models of human cancers because of differences. But I think that it would be a very fruitful approach to cancer research.

There is a good deal of emphasis in cancer research in the area of immunology. So I think we also have to take a look at the immune systems of animals and how they might be utilized in the prevention and control of cancer.

So I think it even goes beyond the area of animal neoplasia per se.

Senator MELCHER. Specifically with Marek's disease and poultry, by finding the presence of a virus and developing a vaccine where the bird developed an immunology, an immune condition against the virus, then that type of leukosis in poultry is inhibited, as you correctly stated.

It does not necessarily guarantee 100 percent immunity, but it is greatly reduced down to a fraction. Then you say that there is no evidence of linking this disease with human infection of cancer, but further studies are probably warranted.

I certainly agree. While the Department of Agriculture, through the Science and Education Administration, has played the leading role in this particular disease, in the development of that vaccine, it is obvious that their funding is very limited.

It is never a surprise to me when one of the agencies come up and testifies and says, "We have *x* number of dollars," in this case specifically $6 million, "that we are utilizing for this type of research, and this type of work, and we think that is adequate."

It is no mystery to me, because through the budget process, no matter who is President, that is what they always have to testify.

So the Office of Management and Budget assesses, or makes a determination, of how much funds are going into the agency, and whenever the testimony before Congress is given by the agency, it is always the testimony really of the Office of Management and Budget, which balances out all of what they do as most significant needs of the Federal funds and where it should be utilized.

Obviously, in your judgment and my judgment, more work is needed. Yet we get that type of testimony from the people we are hoping to direct to do more work and therefore expend more Federal funds for this particular purpose.

I very much agree, doctor, with your summary, and particularly with the point that you express as a concern, that the level of funding proposed in the bill is not adequate to really provide the level of thrust intended in the Animal Cancer Research Act.

It is not the level of funding that I would like to have. It is not enough, but at least it is a start, and if we can have the start, based on the thrust that more basic research is needed, that this is an area that is underfunded, that is, the animal cancer research area is underfunded, and that we can provide more funds very prudently where it is needed for basic research with animals or wildlife, then I think we can perhaps go on from there and build on it.

I certainly agree with your summary, and I want to thank you very much for testifying today and giving us some very excellent testimony for our record.

Dr. SORENSEN. Could I make another observation?

Senator MELCHER. Certainly.

Dr. SORENSEN. You mentioned that additional legislation was needed to provide funds; I agree with that. I am cognizant of the fact that before the animal health research bill there was legislation available to appropriate funds for animal health research, but it just did not get done.

Even though the mechanism exists today for additional animal health research funds, I think there is a lot of merit in Congress specifically targeting funds for animal health research, because then I think something will happen.

It is very difficult to get some of the animal cancer diseases high enough on a priority list so the funds will be directed under the existing mechanism.

Senator MELCHER. That is exactly true, doctor. The argument is made, well; we have an unbalanced Federal budget. The Federal deficits are high, and inflation is worsened because of deficit Federal spending; and therefore we have to have less spending.

That is well and good, but your testimony further—getting away from the basic research aspects of it, just for the purpose of gaining knowledge—your testimony further demonstrates that part of the cost of food is because of the loss of the animals or birds or partial loss caused by the animal not doing well and not producing milk or not gaining weight prior to the time of slaughtering the animal.

Through those losses, we are feeding inflation also. Your testimony has very graphically demonstrated that that is a bigger factor in how we are generating higher prices for animals and birds than a very modest amount annually would be to try to alleviate those losses.

I do not think we do enough to alleviate those

losses, nor do I think we do enough from the basic research aspect of it, just to gain knowledge.

I think we are on very sound ground and very defensible grounds and very prudent grounds, to spend more money here where we know there is not an adequate job being done.

Simply to list four areas of major significance, four or five or six of major significance, that the Science and Education Administration is addressing in their research on animal cancer, poultry cancer, is simply not enough. That in itself is testimony that we are not doing nearly enough.

If we were doing more, these limited benefits we have received so far would be greatly enhanced.

Thank you very much, doctor.

Now we have a panel we are anxious to hear from.

It consists of Dr. Hernan Acevedo, Dr. Michael Naughton, Dr. Myron Blume, and Dr. Vernon Stevens.

STATEMENT OF DR. HERNAN F. ACEVEDO, SENIOR SCIENTIST, DEPARTMENT OF LABORATORY MEDICINE, DIVISION OF EXPERIMENTAL PATHOLOGY, ALLEGHENY GENERAL HOSPITAL, PITTSBURGH, PA.

Dr. ACEVEDO. My main comments here in respect to the bill is in what it refers to in part (d). I was very interested in hearing what my colleagues at the Department of Agriculture research group have been doing. And the main aspect is that the problem of human chorionic gonadotrophin, this material that is also called choriogonadotrophin or CG. We have developed through observations and research here in the United States and in other countries, the concept, since there is enough evidence now that we are dealing with something that we could call a common denominator in respect to the process of malignant transformation occurring in cells of human beings and animals.

Chorionic gonadotrophin is recognized as the hormone of life. It was thought that it was only produced in the human trophoblast. It happens that through investigations at different levels, it appears that this protein is a little bit more ubiquitous, because we have been finding it in cells that are undergoing the process of malignant transformation in different species. Moreover, one of the most important facets of these findings, this material is associated with the cell membrane of the malignant cell. I want to stress again that this does not occur only in human cancers, but also in animal cancers. Perhaps if the chairman permits me, I will give a few slides showing a small part of the research, and after those slides the rest of the panel can make comments.

Senator MELCHER. Certainly.

[Slide presentation.]

Senator MELCHER. Doctor, do I understand that the cells themselves synthesize chorionic gonadotrophin——

Dr. ACEVEDO. Yes; the cells synthesize it for the very simple reason that all the microphotographs that I presented correspond to isolated cell systems, cells in tissue culture.

I did not show slides demonstrating its presence in tissues, because if you show it in tissues, you still can argue about the possibility that the cells from that particular tissue from an entire animal may be taken and/or attaching the material to the cell membranes, that is, the material may have come from other places. Being this tissue culture, we are absolutely sure that the only place where the material can come is from the cell itself, since there is nothing in the culture media analysis performed in the culture media totally negative for the presence of CG-like material.

Therefore, unless the material comes flying in the air, we do not know by which other way it can be present.

Senator MELCHER. Those are cancer cells that you showed, which cells normally would synthesize chorionic gonadotrophin?

Dr. ACEVEDO. The two cells that normally synthesize chorionic gonadotrophin and fix it in their membranes, like the cancer cells, the only two that we know, that we have found are the trophoblasts, of course, and the spermatozoa.

Senator MELCHER. Just those two normally?

Dr. ACEVEDO. Yes. Work done in Texas has corroborated our findings in the spermatozoa. On the other hand, the ovum does not show synthesis; even it has to have the information to synthesize it.

Senator MELCHER. How can you be sure that what you showed on the border of those cells was chorionic gonadotrophin?

Dr. ACEVEDO. Because we are using very specific antibodies against the hormone. The possibility that the reaction could be due to the other product is ruled out because we are dealing with an antibody created to the part of the molecule that is different from luteinizing hormone.

Senator MELCHER. What is your purpose in showing—and I suspect it is—you mentioned the snake cell. Was your purpose to show from snakes or hamsters or other mammals that there is a common agent between mammalian and nonmammalian cancer types of cells?

Dr. ACEVEDO. Yes. It appears that we have in front of us what I would call a common denominator. If we have a common denominator of this type, it looks like we would have to change several aspects in respect to what we think of cancer.

If we have thought that cancer is 300 different diseases, and if we have to make a vaccine out of every one of those diseases that are being induced by different ways, like viruses, chemical compounds and so on, it makes the investigation very expensive and the work very difficult.

But if we have a common compound that is at the level of the cell membrane that have the same immunological activity of chorionic gonadotrophin, and moreover, this compound appears to be a protein of this type, we can think that we have the possibility that we are dealing with one disease that is expressed in 300 different ways.

Senator MELCHER. You are saying that the common denominator is chorionic gonadotrophin?

Dr. ACEVEDO. Or a chorionic gonadotrophin-like material.

Senator MELCHER. Which is a glycoprotein?

Dr. ACEVEDO. It is a glycoprotein because it has biologic activity in people. The jump over the species is even greater because we have found that this material is also present in some bacteria. And these bacterial strains—every time we have found one that expresses the material at the level of the membrane, it is too coincidental that it has always been associated with cancer in human beings.

Senator MELCHER. Now we have discussed somewhat this morning the development of a vaccine for Marek's disease for poultry using a virus which has been successful. How does that use of a vaccine for a specific type of cancer where a virus is involved, as demonstrated in Marek's disease, how does that relate to chorionic gonadotrophin, or does it relate?

Dr. ACEVEDO. It does not relate at all, because with that vaccine you are eliminating the inducer, which is the virus.

Senator MELCHER. In other words, you think that chorionic gonadotrophin might be present and produced in the lymphoids, the malignant lymphoid cells in birds?

Dr. ACEVEDO. If we have the opportunity to study them, I am pretty sure we will find it. We have found it in Rauscher's leukemia, and they all show the same thing.

Senator MELCHER. There may be more questions, but I want to allow the other members of the panel to speak.

Dr. Naughton, I believe you are next.

STATEMENT OF DR. MICHAEL NAUGHTON, UNIVERSITY OF COLORADO HOSPITAL, DENVER, COLO.

Dr. NAUGHTON. I would just like to confirm Dr. Acevedo's observations. We originally came into this field asking the naive question: Why is the placenta not rejected? We started to look at chorionic gonadotrophin, and found the placenta that was covered with it. And at that time there have been some observations that human chorionic gonadotrophin was high in some cancer patients, and we looked at a number of cancers and we found, sure enough, practically all the cells we looked at that were cancers did have the materials on the surface as defined by the antibodies technique.

Senator MELCHER. This probably is not even a question, but let me pursue that for a moment. You identified chorionic gonadotrophin on the placenta of what species?

Dr. NAUGHTON. Humans; this has always been humans.

Senator MELCHER. How did you identify chorionic gonadotrophin on the placenta?

Dr. NAUGHTON. By the immune proxidase system, which is a double antibody technique. You use an antibody directed against the subunit, and you follow this with a sheep antibody that has the proxidase on it. And then the stain shows where the antibodies are localized. And they were localized on the surface of the placenta.

Senator MELCHER. Is that the technique used to

identify chorionic gonadotrophin on malignant cells?

Dr. NAUGHTON. That is exactly the same technique.

Senator MELCHER. What type of malignant cells, again?

Dr. NAUGHTON. All human. We looked at about some 30 tumors, and we only found 2 negatives. What we were calling negatives were cells we could not score.

One was a melanoma that had a brown color to it naturally and couldn't score it positive or negative. The others were negative. It was rather necrotic tissue, so we could not positively identify it.

Since that time, we have extended the investigation.

Senator MELCHER. Are all of these tumors malignant tumors?

Dr. NAUGHTON. Yes.

Senator MELCHER. Please proceed, then. I interrupted you.

Dr. NAUGHTON. It is just a confirmation of what Dr. Acevedo has found.

Senator MELCHER. The difference, perhaps, is that you were working with malignant tumors of animals.

Dr. ACEVEDO. Yes; we have also found the CG-like material in humans' cancers, practically 100 percent of the ones we have examined.

Senator MELCHER. Dr. Blume.

STATEMENT OF DR. MYRON BLUME, MOUNT ZION HOSPITAL, SAN FRANCISCO, CALIF.

Dr. Blume. Let me first identify myself, and tell you what I can testify to and what I can't.

I am a physician and oncologist, specializing in cancer. All of my professional career I have been involved in cancer research, primarily human cancer, and particularly the immunologic aspect of human cancer, what the immune system has to do with cancer, and how it might be manipulated to treat cancer or prevent cancer.

So mainly I am here to answer any questions that the committee might have in regard to the biologic aspects of cancer in humans and experimental animals, and the relationship between animal cancer, animal models of cancer, and human cancer research.

I would like to emphasize at this time that I have not personally done, nor directed any research, concerning the question of human chorionic gonadotrophin, in animal or human cancer, but I am familiar with Dr. Acevedo's work, and I have scrutinized the literature relating to this question.

As far as anything I might say directly related to the legislation under consideration, I think that the veterinarian experts who have already testified are much more qualified than I. Simply from the point of view of a private citizen and a physician, I think that cancer research is not progressing as fast as anyone would like, and I think that additional moneys spent in doing cancer research, be it on animals, domestic animals, farm animals, or experimental animals, can only help the overall progress.

I am sure more money could be spent very effectively. I am sure in particular that more money could be spent more effectively at the basic science level. I think earlier testimony pointed out that it is easy to justify such expenditures, if we spend a million we will save two.

This has been presented by the gentleman from the Department of Agriculture. And I am sure, when dealing with the human situation, one could make the same kind of economic analysis.

If we can prevent or treat more effectively a certain disease, in particular cancer, it would represent an economic saving.

It is much more difficult to justify basic research with that kind of economics. Nevertheless, basic research does need to be done, because the information gained by such research is the foundation of all practical advances in science.

One cannot rely on private industry to carry the burden of basic research because their commitment is more of a pragmatic or practical one. If the problem can be attacked by a trial-and-error method, that is usually what is tried first. There is nothing wrong with that, but sometimes it does not lead to the solutions. Sometimes you have to backtrack. I think that is where we are now in cancer research. I believe we have nearly exhausted the possibilities which can be investigated by trial-and-error. We need more emphasis on basic biological research.

I think also examining in more depth the tumors that occur in farm animals, in domestic animals, pets, and wildlife, is important. The animal models that are conventionally used in cancer research for the most part are very, very highly inbred mice, rats, and guinea pigs, which are susceptible to a variety of induced tumors, induced by chemicals or virus, or "spontaneous" tumors which seem to depend on the inbreeding of the animals for their expression.

I am aware that cattle and livestock are inbred, but not to the extent of the small animals used in laboratory research. In particular mongrel dogs, of which I am very fond, and cats, are much more outbred and the spontaneous tumors that occur in these animals may be a better model for human cancer than some of the models obtained more readily in laboratories.

I think I will stop there and answer any questions that I can.

Senator MELCHER. I am glad you made that point. Because while my background would not lead anyone to believe that my opinion was very weighty on that matter, I have always wondered why the most important medical research we are doing is so much tied up in hamsters, mice, rats and guinea pigs, which seems to me to be, on its face, very little relation to human beings in terms of what the environment is, and particularly the points you make on the inbreeding, very little relationship at all to the environment that man has on this planet, and therefore, probably significantly, the poor types of mammals to be tested to find out what is wrong with me, a different mammal.

Dr. BLUME. Without belittling the gains that have been made, it is very, very apparent that a mouse is not a man. On the other hand, these animals are very easily handled in a laboratory.

Senator MELCHER. They are cheap, too.

Dr. BLUME. They can be dealt with in large numbers and such experimentation is almost always productive of some kind of result which one can then publish, and thereby gain support for one's research. The relevancy of such results to human cancer (or cancer occurring in domestic animals) then remains to be investigated. This method has been fruitful in the past and undoubtedly will be so in the future. I am only suggesting that other approaches and in particular, other animal models may provide additional information.

A human animal is a much more difficult creature to experiment upon. Human material, such as human tumor cells in culture, is much more difficult to use as an experimental model, more time consuming, and less productive of immediate results in terms of treating cancer patients. As a result it has been less successful in competing for the limited funds available.

Senator MELCHER. We mentioned, Dr. Sorensen and I, Jenner, and if he had been working with mice, hamsters, or guinea pigs, I do not suppose we would have smallpox vaccine produced in that generation.

Maybe I am wrong. I am under the impression that laboratory work with mice and rats and guinea pigs is something that has developed in this century, has it not? I cannot recall that Pasteur did much with little rodents, did he?

Dr. BLUME. No; the small laboratory animal certainly has been used much more extensively in this century, and even in the last 50 years.

Senator MELCHER. What Pasteur used to produce his rabies vaccine, wasn't it the spinal column of a goat?

Dr. BLUME. A rabbit.

Senator MELCHER. Thank you very much, Dr. Blume.

Now it is Dr. Stevens.

STATEMENT OF DR. VERNON STEVENS, OHIO STATE UNIVERSITY HOSPITAL, COLUMBUS, OHIO

Dr. STEVENS. First of all, I will identify myself as well.

I am a Ph. D. in reproductive biology. I hold professorships in the obstetrics and gynecology, pathology and zoology departments, and also have major graduate study commitments in veterinarian and agriculture colleges.

I have been studying chorionic gonadotrophin for the last 17 years, and of course, my testimony here is related to that aspect of your bill; although I have certain opinions and thoughts about the other aspects as well.

I have reached the conclusion that chorionic gonadotrophin a long time ago was probably misnamed. As the gentleman from the Department of Agriculture indicated, it is used as a substitute for pituitary hormones in animals to induce ovulation. Therefore, it is a gonadotrophin.

But if one looks at the basic physiology and gets away from the standard textbook definition, you see it does a lot more. I was not at all surprised when Dr. Acevedo found an association with malignant diseases. In our work, which has been primarily aimed at developing a vaccine against chorionic gonadotrophin, it has been shown to be important to the normal acceptance of the placenta quite differently and separately from being a luteinizing hormone in early gestation.

The quantities produced in normal pregnancies cannot be explained by the need for continuing gonadotrophin support of pregnancies.

When we suggested some possible applications, we had the same kind of problems that some of these gentlemen are now having acquiring research funds.

In the sixties, when I was trying to obtain support for developing vaccines against human fertility, the governmental agencies responsible for that kind of research here in Washington practically threw me out of their offices for suggesting such an adventurous idea.

At any rate, I have persisted and have obtained considerable research funds from the World Health Organization, outside this country. We have now successfully developed a vaccine that will prevent fertility based on immunity to chorionic gonadotrophin.

Our research used baboons and chimpanzees. I have been working with, collaborating with, and supporting the efforts of the other gentlemen here interested in cancer research. I have been very sympathetic to their causes and have suggested someone examine the data that they have acquired, listen to the logic, and to consider the direct implications.

I have been very dismayed that they have not been able to acquire significant support for this research. I have talked to many of my colleagues in veterinarian schools about having a vaccine against chorionic gonadotrophin in animals. Their response is that this would probably be damaging to their image as a professional if I were to suggest something so unconventional.

I think the idea of being conservative in our research and to only do a little different than what is the common thing has been a great deterrent to creativity. At the risk of someone funding quacks, agencies have generally waited until a concept is already demonstrated, and then after you have shown it is feasible, they will give you money to dress up your laboratory.

I think the creativity expressed and the courage displayed by these workers to persist in this area of research should be applauded.

Senator MELCHER. Speaking of chorionic gonadotrophin, specifically, while it might be the desire in a species, I think one of the doctors from the Department of Agriculture mentioned sows, in order to bring them into a state of fertility, and therefore enhance the production process for that species, that domestic species of farm animals, is well and good, and he is coming at it from an entirely different point than what you would come at it if you were trying to inhibit fertility.

However, that is also necessary in terms of animals. We would like to inhibit the fertility in dogs and cats, although I have not practiced for 10 years, and I have not paid any attention to what is going on in that field specifically, we are very much interested in doing that.

Can you relate to me any work that has been

done recently using chorionic gonadotrophin to inhibit, prevent pregnancy, for example, in dogs and cats?

Dr. STEVENS. Not chorionic gonadotrophin per se. As one of the gentlemen in the Department of Agriculture explained, biologically chorionic gonadotrophin resembles a luteinizing hormone, and some work has been done at the Colorado State University for immunizing dogs with luteinizing hormones. The antibodies to it suppresses normal pituitary function, and thereby curtail the production of steroid hormones. Thus the heat period, as well as ovulation, is inhibited.

I think that some commercial firms have been interested in their work, and may be pursuing it as a practical product.

Also, there are other areas of work going on to develop vaccines for dogs other than against chorionic gonadotrophin. I think that in this whole area people are reluctant to pursue chorionic gonadotrophin, or as Dr. Acevedo has said, a chorionic gonadotrophin-like substance—a substance associated with a wide variety of malignant tumors—as a vaccine antigen. If you could use an antigen that was a common denominator, then a vaccine would be a very feasible approach.

The normal problem with tumor immunology is, each tumor is biochemically different. And if you had to develop antigens unique to each, it would be very impractical. But this common association of chorionic gonadotrophin with tumors makes it a very appealing approach. It is an across-the-board association, as far as species specificity, then it is applicable to humans as well.

Senator MELCHER. Have you been aware of the work that the Science and Education Administration has been doing on the physiology, what have you, of chorionic gonadotrophin?

Dr. STEVENS. No. I have not been aware of any work that they have done in this area. I do not claim to have followed the history of their funding throughout the years, but in knowing what work is being supported on chorionic gonadotrophin, since that is my field, I have never heard of any specific research grant being awarded to someone from that agency for the study of chorionic gonadotrophin.

Senator MELCHER. Ohio State University is a land-grant college?

Dr. STEVENS. Yes; it is. It has an experimental station associated with it as well in Wooster, Ohio.

Senator MELCHER. And therefore, I guess, that basic research and diagnosis, prevention and control of malignant tumors in animals and birds has not been adequately coordinated.

If chorionic gonadotrophin is involved, as has been demonstrated by Dr. Acevedo's work and others, then I guess this finding is adequate, that there has not been adequate coordination of information that is available.

Specifically, you come from a land-grant college. You have been cooperating with the veterinarians—school of veterinarian medicine there, and the research laboratory connected with the university.

I do not want to belabor the point. It is an obvious fact. There has not been enough coordination or enough money despite however satisfied the Office of Management and Budget is, and the administration, and for that matter, the Department of Agriculture, that $6 million is adequate.

I think it is, on its face, inadequate.

You say you are not surprised. You got some grants not through the National Institutes of Health—is that the agency you were bounced out of?

Dr. STEVENS. I have had several grants from NIH, but not for research in this field.

Senator MELCHER. Specifically, for chorionic gonadotrophin?

Dr. STEVENS. No; what you must do is know what is in vogue in a particular study section. You apply for money for that type of research, not necessarily your best ideas or ones you are most enthusiastic about. You must learn grantsmanship when you become an academic researcher.

I have never acquired 1 dime in 17 years from the Federal Government for research on chorionic gonadotrophin.

Senator MELCHER. But you have from the World Health Organization?

Dr. STEVENS. Yes; I spent over $2 million of their money.

Senator MELCHER. Which is the most generous usually, NIH or the World Health Organization?

Dr. STEVENS. The particular program that supported me is a very small program, about $20 million. The NIH has several billion dollars; of course the pocketbooks are no comparison in size but for chorionic gonadotrophin research, WHO has been far more generous.

Senator MELCHER. The grantsmanship you have

talked about, what is in vogue—what is in vogue in getting grants through NIH?

Dr. STEVENS. In my particular field of reproductive biology, the subject in vogue currently is to study mechanisms of hormone action, hormone receptors, and other basic studies that happen to be the prime interest of certain scientifically politically powerful people in the country.

The kind of research that is supported is the kind that the chairman and the members of the review panel seem to think is important to be done.

There is nothing negative about such work in the sense it is not important. It is just that it is very resistant to new ideas.

I do not mean to be critical of these gentlemen representing the Federal Government, but I think the people involved in the bureaucracy of these funding agencies tend to select people for panels that take conservative approaches to research, and they don't get involved with some people that are reaching too far out for new ideas.

That is what I was referring to concerning a tendency to stifle creativity. It is easy to get money if you want to get on the bandwagon, but if you want to try something different, beyond the usual concepts, then I think you have an uphill struggle.

Senator MELCHER. I believe in May or June of 1978, we asked, here in this very room, we asked Dr. Upton to explain why the peer-review system seemed to be limiting basic research and some of the types we have been speaking about today.

With no reflection on Dr. Upton—after all, he

did not create the peer-review system or the National Cancer Institute. I understand he will be leaving within the next few months to go back, I believe, to the University of New York. Without any reflection on his capabilities, it seems to me that his description of how the peer-review system works in making awards of vast amounts of money was less than satisfactory.

We did ask him specifically at that hearing why he was turning down an application for a grant by Dr. Acevedo as well as some others, and asked him why, just for the sake of basic research, they did not say, go ahead and do it. It is not being done; why not do it?

The answer was that he could not get around the peer-review system.

I think you are right. I think it was obvious then, in this 1978 hearing, that they are so afraid of being criticized for allowing something that was not—I will use your term—that was not in vogue, that they were just afraid to do it.

What happened after that? Did you ever get a grant from NCI?

Dr. ACEVEDO. No. I have not applied again to the NCI because I know I will not get it. I know that a lot of my colleagues have exactly the same experience. In respect to NCI and the National Cancer Act, a tremendous system has been created that is self-perpetuating, and we just look at the amounts of money involved, from approximately $1 billion, 55 percent in 1978, or 1977, 55 percent went only to 20 institutions in the United States; 55 percent.

Senator MELCHER. Of $1 billion?

Dr. ACEVEDO. $900 million or so.

Senator MELCHER. A half-billion dollars went to 20 institutions?

Dr. ACEVEDO. Yes, sir. The system is self-perpetuating. Things happen, for instance, around the National Cancer Act. There has been created some industry-type groups like the Fredricks Cancer Center, in which ex-scientists from the National Cancer Institute work there. According to the rules—I could be wrong, but I think no person from industry can take part in the peer-review system. That is we have persons from these institutions that are supported by grants or contracts from the National Cancer Institute that are part of the peer-review system.

From the American Cancer Society that gets money, $125 to $130 million per year, that is common knowledge, I have received a grant from an American Cancer Society new program. That program is called research development program. They have given me $25,000 for 1 year.

Senator MELCHER. What year was that?

Dr. ACEVEDO. That started November of last year, and it would finish November 30 this year. And they extended it until July, without funds, of course, until my main research grant is re-reviewed again by the American Cancer Society peer review group.

So I have to wait to be funded, if I am funded, until July 1. It is a well-known fact, that one of the high officers of the American Cancer Society is retiring. From there he goes to one of our more-or-less well-known cancer centers, and at the same time that hospital is receiving, and that came out in the cancer letter, a fat amount of American Cancer Society money to continue investigation in that particular institution, medical school.

[The following information was subsequently submitted by Dr. Acevedo:]

[Excerpts from "The Cancer Letter"—Vol. 5, No. 46—pp. 1 and 2, Nov. 16, 1979]

ACS Plans To Award 10 New Institutional Grants For Up To $200,000 a Year in Cause and Prevention

The new special institutional grants announced last week by the American Cancer Society eventually may support long term programs at 10 institutions with up to $200,000 a year each for research on cancer cause and prevention. Funds for the new grants will come from the ACS special donors program and will not be taken from the $44 million traditional investigator initiated grants programs.

The first award under the new program will be to Mount Sinai School of Medicine of the City Univ. of New York, with Irving Selikoff as the principal investigator.

* * *

ACS in 1971 began its support of the Environmental Cancer Research Project, a three way collaborative intramural research venture involving E. Cuyler Hammond and his staff at ACS, Selikoff and staff at Mount Sinai and Oscar Auerbach and staff at the Veterans Administration Hospital in East Orange, N.J. This collaborative research effort will continue but will become incorporated administratively into the special institutional grant award at Mount Sinai.

Hammond, who recently retired as ACS vice president for epidemiology and statistics, will join the faculty of Mount Sinai as director of an epidemiology educational program and will continue as a consultant with ACS. Lawrence Garfinkel has assumed the position of vice president for epidemiology and statistics.

There are three major components to the Mount Sinai special institutional grant—the information unit, the Hammond faculty appointment, and the three way collaborative Environmental Cancer Research Project. The current annual budget will be about $540,000, of which about $190,000 will be from the special donors fund, contributed "generously and perceptively," ACS said, by the ACS Illinois Div. for the first two years of the project. Support of the Environmental Cancer Research Project already comes from regular ACS research funds.

* * *

[Excerpts from "The Cancer Letter"—Vol. 5, No. 46—p. 1, Nov. 16, 1979]

In Brief

Gusberg Heads ACS, With Scanlon as President-Elect; MDA Honors Holland, D'Angio, Landing

Saul Gusberg, chairman of the department of obstetrics and gynecology at Mount Sinai School of Medicine, was installed as president of the American Cancer Society at the organization's annual meeting last week. He succeeds LaSalle Lefall. Edward Scanlon, director of surgical oncology at Northwestern Univ., was elected vice president and president-elect.

* * *

Dr. ACEVEDO. There is sort of a self-perpetuating system that unfortunately has been created, using the crash approach. We can take care of cancer the same way as we took care of going to the

Moon. It is a natural thing when a system like that exists, and cancer centers are created. Besides, scientists, of course, are human beings, and there is perhaps a psychological sort of barrier, sometimes I ask myself—in reality I don't know if I have to say this or not—why kill the goose that lays the golden eggs?

Senator MELCHER. Dr. Naughton?

Dr. NAUGHTON. I have been supported by a grant for perinatal medicine research—I am basically a protein chemist. I am a Ph. D. but I have a joint professorship in obstetrics-gynecology.

Senator MELCHER. Where does that grant come from?

Dr. NAUGHTON. From NIH. I have applied for three major grants since 1975 for research with HCG and have not been funded. I have applied for two minor ones in a block grant which, again, were not funded.

Senator MELCHER. NCI and they have not been granted?

Dr. NAUGHTON. Yes.

Senator MELCHER. Dr. Blume, are you in on this?

Dr. BLUME. I have never applied to do work on HCG. I have had a number of grants turned down by the National Cancer Institute, some of which have been approved and not funded, some have simply not been approved.

It is a well-known fact that the National Cancer Institute itself has stated that they don't get enough money to fund all of the grants that they approve.

At the same time I very much agree with what

Dr. Acevedo said, the grants that are funded generally go to a restricted group of investigators, most of whom sit on the review committees that are part of the peer review system.

So there are very few people that are part of the reviewing process who are not funded by the same process, and vice versa.

Senator MELCHER. I do not want to dwell any longer on the National Cancer Institute and its peer review system. I have made my thoughts known on it to Dr. Upton in the 1978 hearing, and I do not know whether it has improved any. I would hope it has.

What we are really attempting to do in this bill is just get somewhere else, very frankly, and see if by getting somewhere else, it is not constructive and conducive to progress.

I find myself really very—a very poor promoter of the economy when it comes to basic research, particularly in medicine. I encourage basic research; I encourage Federal funds for basic research in medicine.

I do not want to draw the purse strings; I want to open them up. All of us here in Congress, whether in the House or in the Senate, have to justify to our constituents how we can allow problems of the Federal deficit, problems of very worrisome inflation, damaging inflation, by our actions here, specifically, votes on specific appropriations.

We also all have our druthers on where we are going to try to save money and therefore cut the deficit. But I feel that in the case of basic research, whether it is in medicine, or for that matter, agronomy or soil or water pollution or hydrology, particularly in my State in the West, I do not want to draw the purse strings.

My druthers are to make the savings elsewhere. I firmly believe that when we use basic research, we are really attacking the very causes of our problems, including economic problems, inflation, Federal deficits.

We all benefit, and it will not necessarily take very long. It is not like it is somewhere in the next century. It is within the eighties or nineties. It will pay off, better than anything in Las Vegas.

That is my opinion and my judgment, and I am sure that you would echo that.

Dr. Acevedo. I would like to point out that from my point of view, and I think that also from several of my colleagues here, that research on cancer in animals, like cats and dogs, is of the utmost necessity, for the very simple reason, as you pointed out, that when we are working with the usual laboratory animals we are dealing with a very inbred, homogeneous type of animals, and the human being is not homogeneous at all.

In the cat and dog we have no such homogeneity like in the experimental animal. One of the big problems in the area of research in cancer is that everything we do at the level of human beings, we have to wait for 20, 30 years before we see the results.

Here, in place of the human being—we have an experimental animal, animals that we can use, like cats and dogs, in which their lifespan is much shorter, and we can have results of certain types of investigation, for example, effects of vaccines or things like that, that may be extrapolated more easily to the human beings because of their life-spans and heterogeneity.

We can have those observations in a relative short time, where in the human beings we would have to wait 40 years. So that part of the bill is of tremendous necessity. It is very interesting that I have not seen, not at NCI, not at any other level I have known, experiments of this type of basic experimentation in cancer utilizing these various types of domestic animals.

Senator MELCHER. You are echoing the exact point that Dr. Blume made, and the need to look at other species other than just laboratory species.

First of all, I take it that you all feel that there is a possibility of structuring a vaccine. I do not know if that is a good name, but some method of prevention of cancer by pursuing basic research on cancer.

Dr. STEVENS. Absolutely. Of course, as you said, it is premature to say exactly what kind of therapy would be involved, but I think the basic association of chorionic gonadotrophin with all these malignancies will provide some key to an effective therapy.

It should be investigated with high priority.

Dr. BLUME. I would like to modify that by taking a little more cautious stance, without losing any of my enthusiasm for pursuing the investigation of HCG and cancer. I think ever since people started to research cancer, to look at the malignant cell, one of the first questions that has always been asked is: "What makes this cell malignant, and what do malignant cells have in common that normal cells do not have in common?"

There have been a number of different ideas investigated, and none of them have been terribly productive. At the cellular or molecular level no common denominator has been found linking all, or even most malignant diseases. In this regard HCG may be a first.

Whether HCG synthesis is an accident resulting from malignant transformation, or something that caused the malignant transformation, is really not of great importance at this stage of the game.

So the finding so far that HCG or HCG-like material is almost universally present when it is sought for, is a very important observation. I think it cannot help but better our understanding of the malignant process, and the difference between malignant and nonmalignant growth.

The practical application of this information in the treatment or prevention of cancer is something that will take considerably more time to work out. Consequently I would refrain from trying to justify this area of investigation by postulating short-term gains in the treatment of cancer patients.

But I think it certainly needs to be pursued. It is as important, if not more important, than any other area of basic research that is currently being investigated with megabucks, and I think this is something that has been seriously neglected.

Dr. Naughton. I am primarily interested in a reason for it. I think the vaccine is down the road, but I think if you have a reason, then you can logically start the thing.

Dr. Acevedo. As a scientist from the University of Colorado said, if I knew in the research I am going to do what the results are going to be 6 months from now, I will never do research.

Senator MELCHER. We have been talking about chorionic gonadotrophin and possibly identification as a possible agent. How does this fit into diagnosis? We have not talked about that.

Dr. NAUGHTON. I was at a meeting last week in Albuquerque, N. Mex., where they were using antibodies to HCG, and were able to visualize it. The amount of HCG in circulation in the serum, though, did not appear to bear any relationship to HCG presence on the surface of the cell.

There are two things people get mixed up in. The human placenta, for instance, at term, appears to have about the same amount on it as it does in the first trimester, even though the amount that is in circulation is enormous.

I think an explanation has to be sought for this.

Dr. ACEVEDO. We have been looking from two different points of view. One is the immunohistochemistry, that is being used more and more as an aid to the pathologist, because you can do the reactions in frozen sections; and we are working very hard in that aspect, and there are several places that it is being done, in England and Belgium.

There is another aspect that we have also run into. In the blood of patients having cancer that one of my collaborators was looking at, a possibility exists in those individuals where you don't find circulating serum chorionic gonadotrophin. This came up just by a hunch and some rationalization. We took a look at the lymphocytes. When HCG determinations are done in blood, it is done in serum, so the blood is separated.

What we did was the contrary to that. We found in our preliminary studies there was a high percentage of the lymphocytes of cancer patients that attach the material that we are calling chorionic gonadotrophin to their cell membrane. This was done by separating the lymphocytes from the rest of the blood cells, and they're doing the chemistry, and we found that there was a relationship.

It looks like there is a relationship with the stage of the disease, something that did not happen when the correlations were done with the circulating hormones and the amount of tumoral mass. Now there is one, due to that special activity of the membrane, a certain percentage of attachment to the antibody.

In our quantification, by counting the lymphocytes, it comes out that in all the cancer patients we have studied, they show an attachment that was from 10 up to 90 percent over the baseline.

We do not know exactly that what we are looking at is HCG, but we are sure that they are lymphocytes. We think there is a population that concentrates or that attaches the material. You cannot find this when you are looking only at serum.

So, a blind study is being done, without any help from Government agencies, using our own scarce funds, and we will see. We think that there is a big possibility with respect to diagnosis.

The other type of diagnostic use that Dr. Naughton talked about, is the work using tagged antibodies, especially technetium that has a much shorter half-life, therefore is much better for use in human beings. And this looks also, in the hands of the investigators, very, very promising, and I personally think we have there a very useful diagnostic method to be applied practically.

Senator MELCHER. Thank you.

I would like to make as part of the record chapters 4 and 5 of the publication, "The Road Not Taken: Toward a Cancer Vaccine," by Dr. Robert Netterberg and Robert Taylor.[1]

I believe they provide some background information.

I want to thank you all very much for being present today to help us with the hearing. Your testimony has been most helpful in demonstrating the lack of pursuing, with any type of figure at all, this opportunity in basic research.

We would hope to improve on the bill after the hearings today and make some changes in it. One of the changes we probably will make is to make sure that qualified research facilities could be considered by the Science and Education Administration.

Furthermore, I am very much in agreement with the point that Dr. Sorensen made, and I do not think I need to ask any of you about that since the amount of funding is very minimal and it should be increased. I suspect that you would all agree with that.

Thank you all very much. This concludes the hearing today.

---

1. Included in original hearings.

The hearing record will be held open for 10 days for any further testimony.

[Whereupon, at 12:20 p.m., the subcommittee adjourned, subject to call of the Chair.]

APPENDIX

[S. 2043, 96th Cong., 1st Sess.]

A BILL To provide for research in the diagnosis, prevention, and control of malignant tumors in domestic animals, poultry, and wildlife.

Be it enacted by the Senate and House of Representatives of the United States of America in Congress assembled, That this Act may be cited as the "Animal Cancer Research Act".

SEC. 2. Congress finds–

(a) that basic research on malignant tumors or cancers is essential to protect the health of domestic animals, poultry, and wildlife, including birds;

(b) that carcinogenic agents have not been adequately identified in domestic animals, poultry, and wildlife management;

(c) that basic research in diagnosis, prevention, and control of malignant tumors in animals and birds has not been adequately coordinated;

(d) that significant theories of a common factor in malignant tumors, such as chorionic gonadotrophin, have not been pursued in depth; and

(e) that research on diagnosis, prevention, and control of cancer in animals and birds will be beneficial to identify any such common factors in both human and animal malignant tumors, if such exist.

SEC. 3. There is hereby authorized to be appropriated to the Science and Education Administration of the Department of Agriculture $1,500,000 for fiscal year 1980, $3,000,000 for fiscal year 1981, and $5,000,000 annually thereafter for the conduct of basic research on cancer in animals and birds at appropriate facilities within the Department of Agriculture or by grants to other qualified veterinary research facilities.

SENATE COMMITTEE ON AGRICULTURE, NUTRITION, AND FORESTRY STAFF EXPLANATION OF S. 2043

S. 2043 would authorize the appropriation of funds to the Science and Education Administration of the Department of Agriculture for the conduct of basic research on cancer in animals and birds. The research would be conducted at appropriate facilities of the Department of Agriculture *or* by grants to other qualified veterinary research facilities.

Under the bill, the level of funding would be $1.5 million for fiscal year 1980, $3 million for fiscal year 1981, and $5 million for each fiscal year after 1981.

The bill contains Congressional findings that—

(1) basic research on malignant tumors or cancers is essential to protect the health of domestic animals, poultry, and wildlife, including birds;

(2) all carcinogenic agents have not been adequately identified in domestic animals, poultry, and wildlife;

(3) basic research in the diagnosis, prevention, and control of malignant tumors in animals and birds has not been adequately coordinated; and

(4) research on the diagnosis, prevention, and control of cancer in animals and birds will be beneficial in determining whether there are common factors that cause malignancies in both humans and animals.

[The following material was submitted by Senator Melcher and referred to on p. .]

The Road Not Taken: Toward A Cancer Vaccine
(By Robert E. Netterberg, D.D.S., and Robert T. Taylor)

* * *

Chapter Four*

The Fatal Embryonic Hormone

If the persistent scientists we have discussed in previous chapters had not sacrificed time, money, recognition, and even reputation to work on the problem of cancer-connected bacteria, we doubt that the promising discoveries we are about to describe would have been made in our lifetime, or, if made, understood. If, as we believe, the discoveries are among the most important in the history of biological science as well as in cancer research, then the work of these scientists will not have been in vain. Their faith in their work will ultimately be vindicated.

To understand these discoveries, we must again enter the world of normal cells and normal growth.

When the egg and the sperm unite in mammals, the original cell begins to divide, and the new creature, which is to become a human being or an animal, attaches itself to the wall of the uterus by layers of cells known technically as the trophoblast (literally "nourishing growth").

These cells synthesize and secrete a substance with the jaw-breaking name *chorionic gonadotropin* or *choriogonadotropin*, which we will henceforth abbreviate CG. According to evidence now available,[14 23 26 28 29] one of the functions of CG is to protect the embryo, which, be-

*See footnotes at end of chapter.

cause it has chromosomes from the father would be subject to attack as foreign protein. In 1976, this substance was also located in human spermatozoa.[1,6]

From about 1970, different investigators have also found the presence of a CG-like substance in the serum of a great number of patients with cancer,[9,10,22] suggesting that the cancer cells, like the trophoblasts and sperm, are also producers of CG or a CG-like substance. Further studies by investigators at Denver and Pittsburgh[2,30] demonstrated that cancer cells, irrespective of origin, type of cancer and even *species*, do indeed synthesize the CG-like compound. These discoveries vindicate, in a sense, the pioneer scientist Beard,[8] who in 1902 theorized that cancer cells were much like trophoblastic cells.

The mechanism by which CG on the surface of fetal cells, spermatozoa, and cancer cells defends such cells, appears to be physical-chemical in nature. CG, because of the presence in its molecules of a substance called sialic acid, has a high density negative electric charge.[15,24,32,34] Agents of the immune system also carry a negative electric charge, but of lesser magnitude. A very basic principle of electricity states that objects with similar electric charges repel each other, an effect easily demonstrated by the action of small charge foam balls or the leaves of a potentiometer. Indeed, such agents of the immune system such as the white blood cell macrophages cannot get close enough to attack the cancer cell, although the lymphocytes have signaled that the tissue is foreign. Further, some of the immune system white blood cells become coated with CG themselves and this renders them ineffective against the cells, even if they actually touch them.[7] The presence of CG in the cell membrane in quantities large enough to repel the agents of the immune system is a practical definition of malignant transformation or *cancer*.

We have already discussed the long work of Dr. Virginia Livingston-Wheeler in classifying and studying a microbe she has named *Progenitor cryptocides.* In a 1974 issue of the Transactions of the New York Academy of Sciences,[33] Dr. Livingston-Wheeler announced the confirmation of a hunch that the microbe also synthesizes a CG-like material much like the material synthesized by cancer cells. Her observation was confirmed by two other scientists, Drs. Herman Cohen and Alice Strampp of Princeton Laboratories, Inc. in a paper published in 1976.

An extraordinary discovery! Did the scientific world applaud and shout "Eureka!"? Hardly. The announcement fell upon the scientific community with all the clamor of soft snow.

Yet this was the first time that any bacterium had been shown to produce a substance virtually identical to a human hormone, one so similar that only very sophisticated tests could measure any difference. Further, this compound was the same compound synthesized by cancer cells, spermatozoa, and the trophoblast. Obviously, some direct link exists between the bacterial microbes and cancer cells!

Not all scientists ignored this extraordinary discovery. Two alert scientists who did not ignore it were Hernan F. Acevedo and Malcolm Slifkin. Both of them are well known and recognized scientists, members of several of the most prestigious scientific societies, national and international. Dr. Acevedo is the Senior Scientist in the Division of Experimental Pathology of the Department of Laboratory Medicine, William H. Singer Memorial Research Institute of the Allegheny General Hospital, in Pittsburgh, Pennsylvania, which he joined in 1966. Since 1968, he has also held the position of Adjunct Assistant Professor of Microbiology and Cell Biology, Pennsylvania State University. He has been principal author or co-author of more than 100 scientific papers, abstracts, and chapters of books on such diverse topics as hormones in cancer and mesenchymal diseases, pituitary and adrenal dysfunction, biochemistry of reproduction, and hormone metabolism in normal and abnormal tissues.

Dr. Malcolm Slifkin has been the Head of the Section of Microbiology and Immunology, Department of Laboratory Medicine, Allegheny General Hospital since 1964, and Adjunct Professor of Microbiology, Pennsylvania State University since 1965. Since 1975, he is also Clinical Assistant Professor of Pathology, University of Pittsburgh School of Medicine.

Dr. Slifkin is also main author or co-author of many papers in the fields of bacteriology, virology, immunology, and cancer research.

Acevedo and Slifkin wrote the first account of the identification of choriogonadotropin in human spermatozoa.[1] In 1976, they also reported for the first time the synthesis of the CG-like material by cancer cells in tissue culture and from animal models at the Third International Symposium on Detection and Prevention of Cancer, that was held in New York City.[2 30]

One of their most significant publications appeared in the April, 1978 issue of *Cancer*, the official research journal of the American Cancer Society. This was an article entitled "Immunohistochemical Localization of a Choriogonadotropin-like Protein in Bacteria Isolated from Cancer Patients."[3]

This paper contains three important and interesting findings: (a) that fifteen strains of bacteria isolated from tissues of cancer patients show the property of synthesizing a CG-like substance; (b) that the CG-like substance was absent in noncancerous human cells and in bacteria not isolated from cancer tissues; and (c) that the CG-like protein was found on the surface of bacteria and cancerous cells.

In a later scientific paper, published in the June 1979 issue of *Infection and Immunity*, one of the official journals of the American Society of Microbiology, Acevedo,

Slifkin, and associates also described the presence of the CG-like substance in a strain of bacterium called *Eubacterium lentum.*[4] This was the first time that an anerobic bacterium (one that lives without air) has been shown to synthesize the hormone-like substance. Of further interest is the fact that this bacterium was originally isolated in 1938 from a rectal tumor in France! The bacterial strain was obtained from American Type Culture Collection which keeps microbial strains in culture and on file for scientists to utilize in research. This discovery shows that the property of CG-like hormone synthesis is transmitted by the bacterium from generation to generation. This publication further supported the original observation of these scientists that all bacteria exhibiting the CG phenomenon were isolates from a cancer patient, although *not all* bacteria isolated from cancer patients exhibit this ability.

In other writings, these researchers have described that in a manner almost identical to that of cancer cells, the CG-like material is localized in the membranes of the cell wall of bacteria.[31] A further publication by researchers from the Rockefeller University[30] demonstrated that the material isolated from cultures of above-mentioned bacteria possessed the most important characteristic of the hormone, that is, to stimulate the uterus of a rat when injected into a live animal, in other words what scientists call *in vivo* (in life) biological activity.

Acevedo and Slifkin are applying at present for grants (a) to systematically screen bacteria of known origin for the presence of the CG-like hormone, (b) to determine the clinical frequency of the CG-like protein in bacteria isolated from patients with different types and stages of cancer as well as from non-cancerous patients, (c) to study further if any structural differences exist between bacteria that synthesize the CG-like protein and those that do not, and (d) to determine the intracellular location of the CG-like protein.

If it turns out that only bacterial strains that are growing in or have grown in the presence of cancer cells synthesize the CG-like protein, several possible results can follow:

(a) The question of the possibility of a CG-producing bacterium being the *cause* of cancer needs to be reconsidered. As Acevedo writes: "An old area of research will have to be reopened and started with a fresh approach."

(b) The presence of the CG hormone might be an excellent diagnostic tool to detect cancer in early stages.

(c) If CG or the CG-like protein are found *only* in cancer cells, spermatozoa, trophoblasts, and cancer-related bacteria, this would offer a real possibility for developing a cancer vaccine!

The National Cancer Institute has refused grants to Dr. Acevedo and his group to proceed with these studies.

A paper by Canadian researchers Malkin, Kellen, Cameron, and Farber, recently published in the *Scandinavian Journal of Immunology*,[10] reports that CG is present in pre-malignant liver cells in rats, suggesting that the production of CG is part of a "programed phenomenon."

To sum up, these basic discoveries that cancer-related bacteria and cancer cells share this remarkable ability to synthesize CG or a CG-like protein suggests to us some new facts about cancer.

First of all, if it is true that every cancer, whether in the bloodstream, the lymphatic system, or in organs, is producing CG or a CG-like material, then from this standpoint all cancer is *one* disease, not many, as traditional teaching suggests. Of course, it may attack different parts of the body.

Second, the presence of this CG protein in every cancer cell suggests that the mechanism of the cancer cell is *one* mechanism, regardless of the different triggering causes such as carcinogens or radiation.

Third, the presence of the CG protein on the surface of every cancer cell and also on bacteria found in the cancerous tissue (including urine) of cancer patients suggests that *something* connects the two phenomena, although just what the relationship is, is not entirely clear. Dr. Livingston-Wheeler hypothesizes that the bacterium (she still insists that it is one and the same bacterium and that its "filterable phase" may contaminate other bacteria in the cancerous patient) invades the cell and perhaps lies dormant within it. Then some internal or external outside disturbance—chemical or radiation—produces a crisis in the cell and the genetic coding of the invader either begins the synthesis of CG or somehow sets off the latent gene for CG in the cell itself. Another hypothesis suggests that the bacteria takes on the property of synthesizing the CG protein somehow from the cancer cell as *it* becomes a cancer cell.

Fourth, if cancer is one disease, then perhaps by attacking the CG protein, with its heavy negative charge, particularly as this seems to be the mechanism by which cancer avoids the immune system, cancer may be stopped by chemicals that neutralize CG.

This immensely promising line of research, with future possibilities to be discussed more fully in the next chapter, is the direct result of over eighty years of research into cancer-related bacteria, research that has been swept under the rug, denied, and mocked, while thousands of victims have died unnecessarily in the terrible pain of cancer. The implications that lie ahead are incomprehensible when this nation finally does come to the realization of what has happened since 1924.

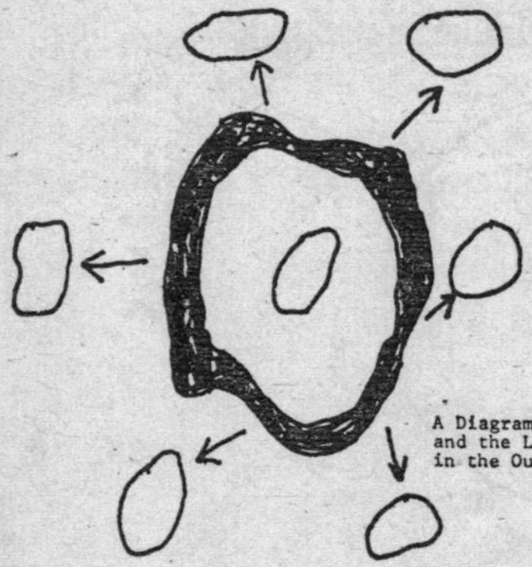

The CG-like hormone (black border) localizes in the outer membrane of the cancer cell and its high negative electric charge wards off white blood cells from approaching and destroying the cell.

A Diagramatic Illustration of a Cancer Cell and the Localization of the CG-like Hormone in the Outer Membrane Wall

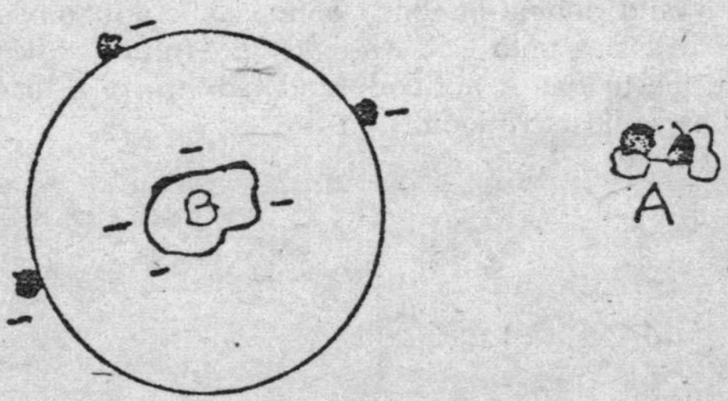

FIGURE A. This represents a classic experiment. Foreign liver cells (A) were immediately attacked and devoured by agents of the immune system (black bodies). The cancer cell (B) is not attacked because the negative charges repel the agents of the immune system at a distance too far for destructive effects to reach the cell.

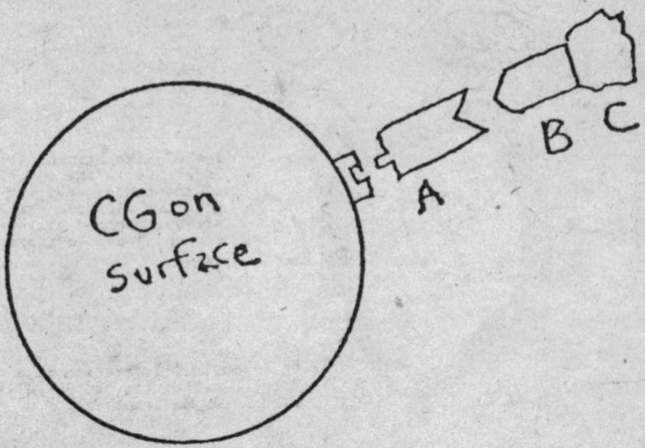

Antibody and double antibody action. The antibody A specifically will lock unto CG. Antibody B (from another animal) is specific to the A antibody and may carry a marker (C) such as radioactive iodine.

CHAPTER FOUR FOOTNOTES

1. Acevedo, H. F., M. Slifkin, G. R. Pouchet, M. Rakhshan. "Identification of the β-subunit of Choriogonadotropin (CG) in Human Spermatozoa" in *The Testis in Normal and Infertile Men,* ed. P. Roen and H. R. Nankin. New York: Raven Press, 1978, pp. 185–192.

2. Acevedo, H. F., M. Slifkin, M. Pardo, G. R. Pouchet, M. Rakhshan. "Human Chorionic Gonadotropin in Cancer Cells. I. Identification in *in vitro* and *in vivo* Cancer-Cell Systems. In *Detection and Prevention of Cancer,* Part 2, Vol. I, ed. H. E. Nieburg, New York: Marcel Dekker, Inc. 1978, pp. 957–963.

3. Acevedo, H. F., M. Slifkin, G. R. Pouchet, M. Pardo. "Immunohistochemical Localization of a Choriogonadotropin-like Protein in Bacteria Isolated from Cancer Patients." *Cancer, 41:* 1217–1229, 1978.

4. Acevedo, H. F., M. Slifkin, G. R. Pouchet-Melvin, E. A. Campbell-Acevedo. "Choriogonadotropin-like Antigen in the Anaerobic Bacterium, *Eubacterium lentum,* Isolated from Rectal Tumor." *Infection and Immunity, 24:* 920–924, 1979.

5. Adejuwon, Christopher, S. J. Segal, S. Mitsudo. "Protease Inhibitor Abolishes the Apparent hCG-like Immunactivity in Human Tissues." Program of the Endocrine society 61st Annual Meeting, June 1979, *Abst. 954.*

6. Asch, R. H., E. O. Fernandez, C. J. Pauerstein. "Immunodetection of hCG-like Substance in Human Sperm." *Fertility and Sterility, 28:* 1258–1262, 1977.

7. August, Charles, S. Cox, M. Naughton. "Resistance of Cultured Choriocarcinoma Cells to Cell-mediated Cytotoxicity of Mitogen-Activated Lymphocytes." *Journal of Clinical Investigations, 63:* 428–436, 1979.

8. Beard, J. "Embryological Aspects and Etiology of Cancer." *Lancet, 1:* 1758, 1902.

9. Beck, J. S., I. B. Porteous, J. L. Ullyot, "Gonadotropin Secreting Bronchial Carcinoma: Aberrant Endocrine Activity or Trophoblastic Differentiation?" *Journal of Pathology, 101:* 59-62, 1970.

10. Braunstein, G. D., J. L. Vaitukaitis, P. P. Carone, G. T. Ross. "Ectopic Production of Human Chorionic Gonadotropin by Neoplasms." *Annals of Internal Medicine, 78:* 39–45, 1973.

11. Braunstein, G. D., V. K. Kamdar, J. Kanabus, J. Rasor. "Properties of Human Chorionic Gonadotropin Produced *in vi-*

tro by Ovarian Carcinoma Cells." *Journal of Clinical Endocrinology and Metabolism, 47:* 326–332, 1978.

12. Chou, Janice Y., S.-S. Want, J. C. Robinson. "Regulation of the Synthesis of Human Chorionic Gonadotropin by 5-Bromo 2'-deoxyuridine and Dibutyrl Cyclic AMP in Trophoblastic and Nontrophoblastic Tumor Cells." *Journal of Clinical Endocrinology and Metabolism, 47:* 46–51, 1978.

13. Cohen, H., A. Strampp. "Bacterial Synthesis of Substances Similar to Human Chroionic Gonadotropin." *Proceedings of the Society of Experimental Biology and Medicine, 152:* 408–410, 1976.

14. Comings, David. "Lymphocyte Transformation in Response to Phytohemagluttinin During and Following a Pregnancy." *American Journal of Obstetrics and Gynecology, 97:* 213–217, 1967.

15. Defendi, V. G. Gasic. "Surface Mucopolysaccharides of Polyoma Virus Transformed Cells." *Journal of Cell Composition Physiology, 62:* 23–26, 1963.

16. Fauve, Robert M., B. Hevin, H. Jacob, J. Gaillard, F. Jacob. "Antiinflammatory Effects of Murine Malignant Cells." *Proceedings of the National Academy of Science, 71:* 4052–4056, 1974.

17. Fontain, Yves-Alain, E. Burzawa-Gerard. "Esquisse de L'Evolution des Hormones Gonadotropes et Thyreotropes des Vertebres." *General and Comparative Endocrinology, 32:* 341–347, 1977.

18. Ghosh, Ninaik, A. Rukenstein, R. P. Cox. "Induction of Human Choriogonadotropin in HeLa-Cell Cultures by Aliphatic Monocarboxylates and Inhibition of Deoxyribonucleic Acid Synthesis." *Biochemical Journal, 166:* 265–274, 1977.

19. Malkin, A., J. A. Kellen, A. Kolin, R. Cameron, E. Faber. "The Immunohistochemical Detection of Chorionic Gonadotropin in Experimental Rat Hepatomas." *Scandinavian Journal of Immunology, 8* (sup. 8): 603–607, 1978.

20. Maruo, T., H. Cohen, and S. S. Koide: "Studies on Choriogonadotropin From a Microorganism." Program of the Endocrine Society, 61st Annual Meeting, June 1979, *Abst. 951.*

21. McManus, L. M., M. A. Naughton, Q. Martinez-Hernandez. "Human Chorionic Gonadotropin in Human Neoplastic Cells." *Cancer Research, 36:* 3476–3481, 1976.

22. Muggia, F. M., S. W. Rosen, B. D. Weintraub, H. H. Hansen. "Ectopic Placental Proteins in Nontrophoblastic Tumors: Serial Measurements Following Chemotherapy." *Cancer 36:* 1327–1337, 1976.

23. Pattillo, Roland A., M. R. Facog, M. R. Shalaby, R. O.

Hussa, O. P. Bahl, R. F. Mattingly. "Effect of Crude and Purified hCG on Lymphocyte Blastogenesis." *Obstetrics and Gynecology, 47:* 557–561, 1976.

24. Pattillo, Roland A. "Trophoblastic Cancers: Chorionic Gonadotropin Hormone Production, Antigenic Expression, and Trophoblastic Redifferentiation in Multiple Forms of Malignancy." *Pathology Annual.* New York: Appleton Century Crofts, 1973.

25. Quinones, Jose, G. Mizejewski, W. H. Beierwaltes. "Choriocarcinoma Scanning Using Radio-labeled Antibody to Chorionic Gonadotropin." *Journal of Nuclear Medicine, 12:* 69–72, 1970.

26. Ross, Griff. "Clinical Relevance of Research in the Structure of Human Chorionic Gonadotropin." *American Journal of Obstetrics and Gynecology, 29:* 795–808, 1977.

27. Schlegal-Haueter, Susenna, E., J. C. Robinson, Janice Y. Chou. "Characterization of Human Chorionic Gonadotropin Synthesized by Human Cell Lines." Program of the Endocrine Society 60th Annual Meeting, June, 1978, *Abst. 43.*

28. Segal, Sheldon. "Immunological Methods to Prevent Pregnancy: An Editorial Comment." *Contraception, 13:* 124–127, 1976.

29. Simmons, Richard, V. Cruse, D. G. McKay. "The Immunological Problem of Pregnancy." *American Journal of Obstetrics and Gynecology, 97:* 218–230, 1967.

30. Slifkin, M., H. F. Acevedo, M. Pardo, G. R. Pouchet, M. Rakhshan. "Human Chorionic Gonadotropin in Cancer Cells, II. Ultra-structural Localization." In *Detection and Prevention of Cancer,* Part 2, vol. I, ed. H. E. Nieburgs. New York: Marcel Dekker, 1978, pp. 965–979.

31. Slifkin, M., M. Pardo, G. R. Pouchet-Melvin, H. F. Acevedo. "Immuno-electron Microscopic Localization of a Choriogonadotropin-like Antigen in Cancer-Associated Bacteria." In Press. *Oncology,* 1979.

32. Van Beek, W. P., L. A. Smets, P. Emmelot. "Changed Surface Glycoprotein as a Marker of Malignancy in Human Leukemic Cells." *Nature,* 253: 457–460, 1975.

33. (Wheeler) Wuerthele-Caspe Livingston, Virginia, A. M. Livingston. "Some Cultural, Immunological, and Biochemical Properties of Progenitor Cryptocides." *Transactions of the New York Academy of Sciences, 36:* 569–582, 1974.

34. Whyte, A., Y. W. Loke, "Increased Sialylation of Surface Glyopeptides of Human Trophoblast Compared with Fetal Cells from the Same Conceptus." *Journal of Experimental Medicine, 148:* 1087–1092, 1978.

Chapter Five*

Why We Can Have a Universal Cancer Vaccine

As we have said, cancer experts have long held to the belief that there are many forms of cancer. Some believe that these forms may number as many as 300. They also believe that each of these forms of cancer is a completely different disease rather than one disease. The malignant cells of one form, they say, have nothing in common with cells of another form. For example, leukemia is cancer of the blood forming tissues, but leukemia itself is subdivided into several different types. Carcinomas are cancers of the epithelial cells such as the skin, breast, or the cells that line the stomach. Sarcomas are cancers of connective tissue cells like muscle, fat tissue, or lymph glands.

"Scientific authorities," therefore, have consistently reported to the news media and the public that there can be no "magic bullet" to cure or prevent cancer because we are dealing with many diseases under the heading of the word *cancer*. According to this line of thinking, cancer is not a specific disease like tuberculosis or leprosy.

With the discovery that CG is found on the surface of all cancer cells thus far tested, both animal and human, this long-expounded theory of the cancer establishment—that cancer has various forms or that it is many diseases—literally goes out the window. In reality, the discovery and demonstration of the CG hormone provides for the first time in history a common biochemical denominator for all cancer cells.

So cancer can now be looked upon not as many diseases, but one disease with 300 clinical manifestations, which exhibit themselves as "forms." We can explain fur-

*See footnotes at end of chapter

ther by an example. Tuberculosis is caused by one bacterial microbe, *Mycobacterium tuberculosis*. However, the disease can be located on the skin, lung, or other organs of the body, like cancer. Tuberculosis of the adrenal glands, for example, the classical form of a disease, is called Addison's Disease. These are clinical manifestations or different forms of the same bacterial disease—tuberculosis.

CG is technically what we call an *antigen*. An *antigen*, by definition, is any substance that stimulates the production of antibodies or reacts with them. Antibodies are biological protein substances that "lock on" to that particular antigen associated with bacteria responsible for the disease and stop them from producing their harmful disease effects. They also attack any foreign protein—a reason for rejection of skin grafts or organ transplants. The antigen-antibody reaction is the basis for all vaccines from polio and measles to tetanus. The Salk polio vaccine, a typical example, is made by what is known as attenuation of the polio virus. The polio virus cultures are killed by chemical solutions like carbolic acid or formalin. The Sabin polio vaccine is prepared in a different manner by using for the vaccine live virus which has been weakened by other methods of preparation.

Because CG seems to be a universal antigen, then the possibility of a universal vaccine automatically exists.

The whole purpose of any vaccine is to stimulate specific antibody formation by the immune mechanism of the individual against a particular agent—an antigen. The same antibody development sometimes results when the person acquires the disease. Vaccination is a shortcut to the antibody-development process. The immune system produces specific antibodies against a disease without causing the disease. Antibodies of one disease do not protect against another disease because these are highly specific reactions.

In cancer, an additional promising fact about the CG hormone being synthesized by the cancer cell is its localization in the outer wall membranes of the cell (see diagrams), since this increases its vulnerability to be attacked.

Myron Blume, M.D., Ph.D., Director of the Immunology Center at Mount Zion Hospital in San Francisco, California, and an expert in the field of oncology (tumors) and immunology has this comment:

"The presence of a universal marker, one that is confirmed, will allow us to take a big step in the right direction. If that turns out to be true, it will be the first time, in my vocabulary, what could be called a breakthrough has happened in cancer in the last forty years. If you can prove that every single human cancer cell synthesizes CG, I think that would be very significant."

This statement is in reference to the already existent cancer cell, which the white blood cells cannot attack, not because they are not alerted to do so, but because they cannot approach to attack. The cancer cell must be disarmed by removing the CG hormone shield from the outer border of the cell, because the CG functions somewhat like an electric fence warding off the killer white blood cells.

We should make it clear at this point that if the outer membrane of the cancer cell can be destroyed, the cell cannot survive. This principle applies to any type of cell, normal or cancer.

Further, if the CG synthesis is a normal function in the development of the cancer cells, then obviously its formation can be prevented from happening in the first place. As we have pointed out, once the CG synthesis begins to take place in a cell, and becomes concentrated on the cell membrane, the malignant process is underway. The cells have returned to a primordial or underdeveloped stage and divide completely unchallenged by the body's immune system if they accumulate or utilize the hormone in their membranes. The killer capacity of the immune mechanism of white blood cell response has been neutralized by this hormone.

How would the proposed cancer vaccine work? Thus far, Dr. Virginia Livingston-Wheeler and Dr. Hernan F. Acevedo, working independently in different parts of the nation, have shown that bacteria isolated from cancer patients are also synthesizing CG. Because the microbes share what is known in immunology as common antigenic determinants with the cancer cells, namely the CG-like substance, selected strains of these bacterial microbes can be used as the basis for the preventive vaccine. Hopefully, specific antibody formation will therefore prevent a normal cell from undergoing malignant transformation.

To some degree, antibodies are constantly being formed by the body against normal CG, even though it is a natural body substance, but these are antibodies with very low affinity, meaning the amount of reaction is negligible.[6] Now, because of CG-producing bacteria, the potency can be raised to produce antibodies that will really do the job necessary and with the power required for immunity protection.

Dr. Acevedo has said that we can never stop the cell from its attempt at CG production because cancer is a part of life. But with the production of specific antibodies by vaccine innoculation against these microbes, the malignant transformation process by the cells will be stopped in its tracks from becoming a clinical manifestation, that is, the formation of deadly tumors and lesions which spread and kill. We will, in essence, be attacking and preventing cancer at its very roots. We will be preventing the survival of malignant cells after the cellular transformation has occurred, therefore eliminating the presentation of the clinical disease we call cancer.

No more blind shotgun approach of chemotherapy or deadly radiation in the futile attempt to try and kill cancer cells resulting in torturous and toxic effects to the already cancer-weakened patient. No more attacking an enemy cell which is not understood, because we now know how it functions in its sinister way, being closely and ironically linked to life itself. Cause and effect arguments are no longer important. Because of the universal CG hormone antigen, it does not matter how the cancer was produced, or as the NBC Nightly News reported on December 1, 1977, the antigen can be demonstrated by cancer cells regardless of how the malignant transformation was caused. It does not matter whether it was caused by chemical or viruses. It is always present!

Dr. Acevedo has also had much experience in the field of human reproductive biochemistry. He feels that we may have not only a universal vaccine against cancer but also a vaccine against pregnancy. CG hormone is normally present, as we have shown, in the embryonic trophoblast and male sperm cells. If the vaccine works in preventing a cancer cell from developing, we must entertain the possibility that the CG hormone protection of the trophoblast and of the sperm cells will be destroyed upon administration of the bacterial cancer vaccine. Antibodies against a developing cancer cell would have the effect of destroying the trophoblast or preventing fertilization by destroying the sperm cell's potential.[3] As a matter of fact, in a series of reports of studies in India and reported in the February, 1976, issue of *Contraception*,[1] it was shown that a vaccine that neutralized the biological activity of CG significantly lowered the fertility of female rhesus monkeys. The immunization against human CG was obtained with a conjugate of beta subunit of CG and tetanus toxin. A preliminary report of this work was published in the January, 1976 issue of the *Proceedings of the National Academy of Sciences.*[4]

To many, a pregnancy vaccine may be a Godsend in itself. But if everyone took the cancer vaccine early, then the human race could possibly become extinct. How would this problem be solved? Neither Dr. Acevedo nor

Dr. Livingston-Wheeler or other investigators see this as a serious problem. 90% of all human cancers occur after the age of 40. For those who wish to have children, the obvious solution would be to take the vaccine after age 40, because generally that is past the age people usually have children. The question arises, however, as to how many people would want to take that risk. Have children in the hope of not developing cancer or take the vaccine before the age of 40 and not have children? Before anyone becomes too concerned, we must look at some other possibilities for the future.

Various vaccines, such as the tetanus vaccine, proven effective in preventing diseases, do not provide a lifetime protection. If the cancer vaccine is a type requiring periodic shots to maintain immunity against the cellular process, then the matter of pregnancy can be regulated. Dr. Acevedo believes that we will probably need a booster type of vaccine for cancer with periodic renewal of immunity.

A study by Florence B. Seibert and Robert L. Davis of the Veterans Administration of Bay Pines, Florida, further supports the idea that the vaccine will need boosters. In a report in the *Journal of the Reticuloendothelial Society*, April 1977,[3] they discuss the use of a heat-killed vaccine made from a filterable bacterial strain isolated from a mouse breast tumor. This vaccine depressed the incidence of spontaneous breast cancer about 20% from 39 to 58 weeks. However, about the 60th week, the effect weakened rapidly, so that by the 72nd week, incidence of cancer in vaccinated and control mice was about the same.

On the basis of some studies, critics of the CG proposal have felt that the substance might also be present in normal tissues. Should this be the case, then a vaccine against the CG synthesis could cause harm or destroy normal and vital tissues. However, most recent studies suggest that the substance which reacted in their experiments was not genuine CG or a CG-like substance but rather a common body protease that can mimic CG in certain concentrations and certain diagnostic methods.[5] Therefore, the opposition has lost their final argument when it comes right down to the demonstration of scientific facts.

In light of the CG-like substance produced by the microbes and cancer cells, the possibility of cancer being a low grade contagious disease must be considered (also dismissed as nonsense by the cancer establishment in the past) as evidenced by the leukemia outbreaks in high schools in New Jersey and the epidemic levels of cancer in China and elsewhere in the world.

CHAPTER FIVE FOONOTES

1. Papers from Scientists of the All India Institute of Medical Sciences, *Contraception, 13:* 131–268, 1976.

2. Siebert, Florence B., R. L. Davis. "Delay in Tumor Development Induced with a Bacterial Vaccine." *Journal of the Reticuloendothelial Society, 21:* 279–282, 1977.

3. Stevens, Vernon C. "Immunization of Female Baboons with Hapten-Coupled Gonadotropins." *Obstetrics and Gynecology, 42:* 496–506, 1973.

4. Talwar, G. P., N. C. Sharma, S. K. Dubey, Mr. Salahuddin, C. Das, S. Romarishnan, S. Kumar, V. Hingorani. "Isoimmunization Against Human Chorionic Gonadotropin with Conjugates of Processed β-subunit of the Hormone and Tetanus Toxoid." *Proceedings of the National Academy of Sciences, USA, 73:* 218–222, 1976.

5. Maruo, Takesi, S. J. Segal, S. S. Koide. "Studies on the Apparent Human Chorionic Gonadotropin-like Factor in the Crab *Ovalipes ocellatus.*" *Endocrinology, 104:* 932–939, 1979.

6. Wass, M., K. McCann, K. D. Bagshawe. "Isolation of Antibodies to hCG/LH from Human Sera." *Nature, 274:* 368-370, 1978.

About the Authors

Dr. Netterberg is a 1955 graduate of Saint Louis University School of Dentistry. From 1955 to 1957 he served as a dentist in the U.S. Air Force. He has been in practice in Butte, Montana since 1957. In 1958, he became interested in the work that Dr. M. J. Scott had announced in the 1920s while he was chief of staff of surgery at St. James Hospital, Butte, Montana, when Dr. Scott's early plight was called to his attention by a Catholic priest friend. Dr. Netterberg decided to investigate Dr. Scott's claims and brought him back to Butte from Seattle, Washington where he was living as a poor man.

Proceeding cautiously and thoroughly, Dr. Netterberg then launched somewhat of a side career as an investigative reporter, piecing together in chronological order the work of all of the early scientists presented in this book after spending months and years putting all of it together to the present developments on the bacterial microbes of cancer. In 1977, he took the entire story to NBC News. After six months of checking out the data, the NBC Nightly TV News devoted all of Segment Three in presenting the basic breakthrough for one universal preventive cancer vaccine.

Robert T. Taylor is an associate professor in the Humanities and Social Sciences Department of Montana College of Mineral Science and Technology.

After two years of study of science and mathematics at Montana School of Mines, he transferred to the University of Montana, where he was granted a B.A. (with honors) in 1951 and an M.A. in 1952, both in English. Further education has included graduate study at the universities of Wisconsin and Washington.

For three years, he was the editor of a regional arts magazine and has published thirty-seven articles, poems, and stories, as well as one book, *A Community Symphony Handbook* (1972). In 1969 he won the Mary Brennen Clapp Memorial Poetry Prize.